# PRO
# Nail Care

# PRO
# Nail Care

Salon secrets of the professionals

Leigh Toselli

FIREFLY BOOKS

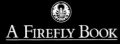

# A FIREFLY BOOK

Published by Firefly Books Ltd. 2009

First printing 2009

Publisher Cataloging-in-Publication Data  (U.S.)

Tosselli, Leigh.

PRO Nail Care: Salon secrets of the professionals / Leigh Tosselli

Includes index

Summary:  A complete guide to the skills and tricks essential to having gorgeous nails. Step-by-step instructions to basic nail care and applying polish. Also included are sections on healthy nails and
nail art.

ISBN-13: 978-1-55407-478-5

ISBN-10: 1-55407-478-9

1. Nails (Anatomy)—Care and hygiene.  I. Title.

646.7/27 dc22   RL94.T6774  2009

Library and Archives Canada Cataloguing in Publication

Toselli, Leigh

Pro Nail Care: Salon secrets of the professionals / Leigh Toselli.

Includes index.

ISBN-13: 978-1-55407-478-5

ISBN-10: 1-55407-478-9

1. Nails (Anatomy)--Care and hygiene.  2. Beauty, Personal.

I. Title.

TT958.3.T67 2009          646.7'27          C2009-903185-X

Published in the United States by
Firefly Books (U.S.) Inc.
P.O. Box 1338, Ellicott Station
Buffalo, New York 14205

Published in Canada by
Firefly Books Ltd.
66 Leek Crescent
Richmond Hill, Ontario L4B 1H1

Conceived, designed, and produced by
Quintet Publishing Limited
6 Blundell Street
London N7 9BH, UK

Project Editor: Asha Savjani
Photographer: Patrick Toselli
Illustrator: Bernard Chau
Designer: Anna Gatt
Additional Text: Sula Paolucci
Editorial Assistant: Tanya Laughton
Art Editor: Zoe White
Art Director: Michael Charles
Managing Editor: Donna Gregory
Publisher: James Tavendale

Printed in China

# CONTENTS

# INTRODUCTION

As well as using our hands for all sorts of practical tasks, we also use them as a way of expressing ourselves and emphasizing what we're saying. They're one of the first things people notice, which is why we need to make the most of them. Beautifully manicured and maintained nails are much-prized attributes that speak volumes about your health and grooming, not to mention your attention to detail.

Neglected hands certainly create a poor impression: bitten nails or torn cuticles indicate a lack of confidence, while perfectly manicured hands suggest somebody who pays attention to detail and takes pride in their appearance.

Everyone can have great looking hands with basic care, meticulous grooming, and regular visits to a professional manicurist. Here they will be buffed, trimmed, softened, painted and filed, massaged and lathered, sloughed, primped, and preened over. Never before has such a variety of artificial nail products been available to extend, repair, or even just strengthen the nail plate, nor has there ever been such a selection of possibilities for adornment, from creative coloring, transfers, and stencils, to rhinestones and gems.

Manicurists and pedicurists are now focused on a lot more than just the natural nail. These days they need to be fully versed nail technicians, conversant in advanced nail technologies and methods, creativity and artistry, business management, and so much more. One of the fastest-growing segments in the beauty business, the nail industry is constantly evolving with new technologies, techniques, and products continually being introduced, providing the nail technician with so much more to ensure the luxury of beautiful nails.

Once you know how to take care of your nails, it will be easy to maintain healthy nails. Beautiful, healthy nails require only a little regular TLC—it needn't be as complicated as you might think. Nails are usually their healthiest in their natural state, requiring a bit of nail polish for protection and regular applications of hand cream as a moisturizer. Allow time for a home manicure every 7 to 14 days with weekly time for touch-ups. Regular home manicures will protect your nails and help improve your image. Good grooming is essential for keeping and maintaining your hands and feet in prime condition.

# Starting at the tips

- After your bath is the ideal time to gently push your cuticles back with a towel, as the warm water will have softened them.
- The cuticle protects the nail root from bacteria. Instead of cutting the cuticle, push it back gently with an orangewood stick or rubber-tipped cuticle-pusher. Strong cuticle growth can be controlled with a cuticle softener or cuticle remover liquid.
- Don't pull or tear hangnails. Cut the flap of skin at the base with clippers or small scissors, and leave the cuticle as intact and untampered with as possible.
- Keep fingernails and toenails at a sensible length. Never clip nails to shorten them. Use an emery board to file nails down to size, but file only when your nails are dry and free from cream.
- Filing straight up against your nail can peel the tip; you should hold the emery board at a 45-degree angle under the free edge of the nail while filing.
- Brittle, peeling nails are caused by dryness. Try to apply a moisturizer or cuticle cream every time you wash your hands.
- Manicure your nails fully approximately every 7 to 14 days, reapplying nail polish as often as necessary.
- Exfoliate them regularly to remove dead skin cells and apply hand cream every time you wash your hands—keep tubs of cream handy next to the sink.
- Always wear rubber gloves when submerging your hands in water, working with hazardous chemicals, or doing messy work like gardening. Try applying your favorite moisturizer before putting on the gloves; the heat from the warm water will help your skin absorb the moisture and treat your hands.
- A base coat is a good investment. Although it is formulated to help nail polish last longer, it also helps prevent colored polish from staining your nails.

- Use nail polish remover as infrequently as possible—especially those containing acetone, as they tend to dry nails out. Use a minimal amount on the nail and avoid getting too much onto the cuticle and skin.
- Never peel or scrape off nail polish or use metal instruments on the nail surface to push back the cuticles, unless you're a professional and know what you're doing. This can scrape off the protective cells of the nail surface. Peeling off flaking nail enamel is also very damaging.
- Avoid using your nails as tools. Instead, keep a screwdriver handy; it'll prolong the life of your manicure.
- Change footwear often and avoid wearing the same pair of shoes every day. It is as important to care for your feet as it is your hands.
- Keep your nails out of your mouth! Biting nails can damage the nail and the cuticle, leading to the transfer of harmful organisms to the nail, which can result in infection.
- When faced with repetitive tasks, take time out to wriggle your hands and fingers, wrists, and arms, to maintain a normal range of movement and to help prevent Occupational Overuse Syndrome.

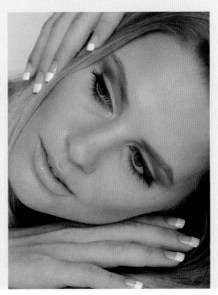

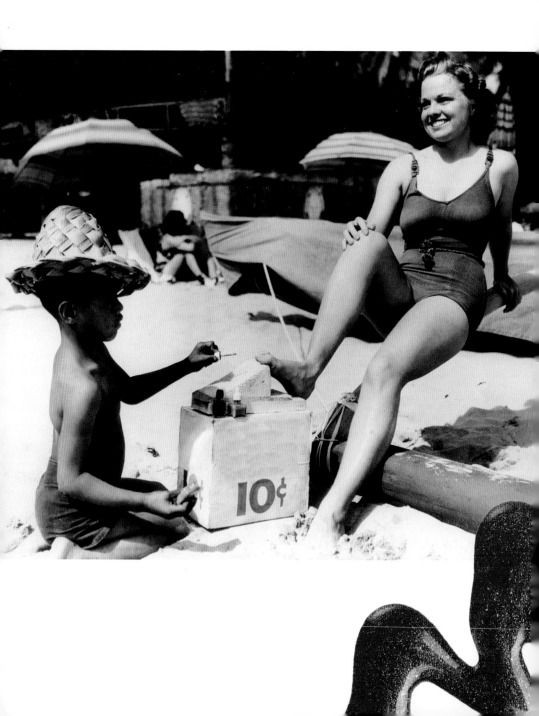

# A HISTORY OF NAIL CARE

Manicured nails can be traced back some 4,000 years to southern Babylon, where noblemen used solid gold implements to manicure their nails.

Manicure instruments have also been found in Egypt's royal tombs. Body decoration, including henna as a stain for fingernails and toenails, has been practiced across the world for centuries. The Egyptians used nail color to signify social order—they used reddish brown stains derived from the henna plant to color their nails as well as the tips of their fingers, with shades of red being the most desired. Queen Nefertiti, wife of King Akhenaton, colored her fingernails and toenails ruby red; Cleopatra favored deep rust red. Women of lower rank who colored their nails were permitted only pale hues. The Chinese used a combination of Arabic gum, egg whites, gelatin, and beeswax to create their colored lacquer. They also used a mixture of pulped rose for color, or orchid and impatiens petals combined with alum, which, when applied to nails overnight, left a pinkish, reddish stain. The Incas could well have been the first to introduce nail art; their fingernails were decorated with pictures of eagles.

Aristocrats grew their nails up to almost 10 inches long as a sign that they performed no manual labor and to indicate their wealth and privilege. Great care was taken to protect each nail; they were often encased in silver or gold sheaths lined with soft padded silk. During the Chou Dynasty of 600 BCE, Chinese royalty often chose gold and silver, and black and red to enhance their nails—colors that would differentiate them from ordinary women. Lower-class women had to be content with lighter shades and if non-royalty were seen sporting the "royal colors," they could be executed. But women weren't the only ones being manicured. In both Rome and Egypt, commanders in the military painted their nails to match the color they wore on their lips, before heading into battle.

The French manicure made its first appearance in eighteenth-century Paris. Its signature white tips and natural pink base found favor in the French court and, years later, were revived in the 1920s and 1930s. By the turn of the nineteenth century,

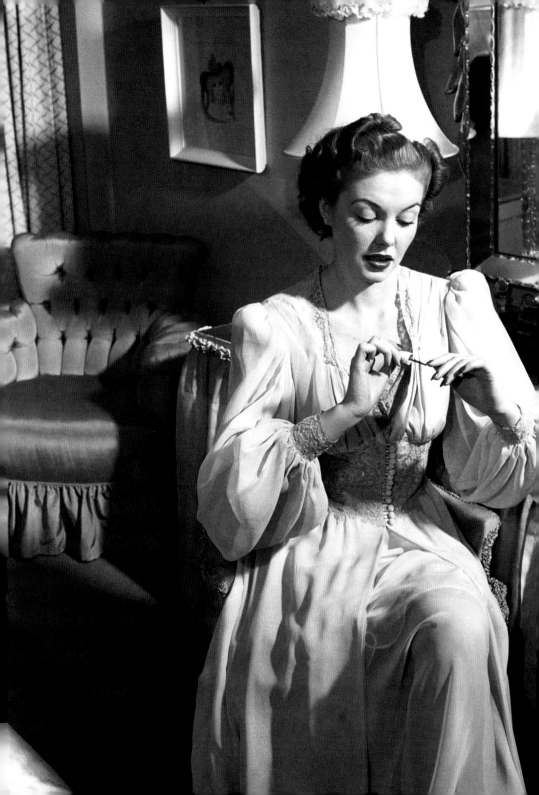

nails were being tinted with scented red oils, powders, and creams, and polished or buffed with a chamois cloth rather than being simply painted.

After World War I there was a surplus of leftover nitrocellulose, which had been used for military explosives. By trial and error, it was discovered that boiling nitrocellulose made it soluble in organic solvents, which, once evaporated, resulted in a glossy, hard lacquer. Around 1920, the automobile industry became interested in developing this lacquer for painting assembly line cars— nitrocellulose lacquer was the paint used by Ford Motors. Not long afterward, Michelle Ménard, who is credited with inventing nail lacquer, refined the lacquer formula by adding softening resins to the basis for nail polish, inspiring the introduction of colored nail enamels.

Nail polish, as we know it, is a twentieth-century phenomenon. In 1917, Cutex introduced the first tinted liquid nail polish, made from natural resins colored with dyes. Technology developed, and the 1920s saw nail polishes made from plasticized nitrocellulose, but this formula didn't adhere well to the nail and wore off quite quickly. In 1929, perfumed polish was introduced, but its popularity was short-lived. In the 1930s, Revlon introduced a revolutionary opaque nail enamel with a creamier coverage and special color pigments, and a year later the company introduced coordinating lipstick and nail colors. In 1938, manicures cost from 25 cents to $3.50 in the U.S., depending on whether or not polish was being applied. The screen-sirens of the 1950s were popularizing bold nail colors and by the 1960s, pale nails were all the rage. Mary Quant launched her first makeup range with six nail colors in 1965, and Boots 17 nail varnish was launched in 1968 with a revolutionary non-drip formula.

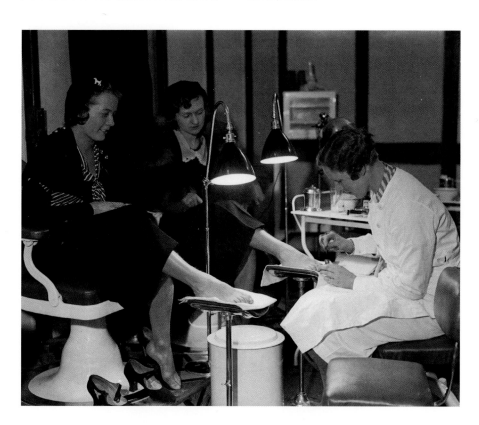

The initial concept of artificial nails came from the dental industry, as dental technicians started playing around with the polymers and adhesives that they used to create crowns, molds, and other dental applications. These materials could be used to create strong solid structures that could go into the mount, and before long, they realized they could use these to lengthen and protect the nails. The earliest resultant artificial nails used a monomer and polymer mix, applied to the nail and extended over a supporting form. As this hardened, the form was removed and a natural extension of the nail plate was achieved. Today, our fascination with beautiful hands and nails continues to grow, resulting in the multibillion dollar industry seen worldwide today.

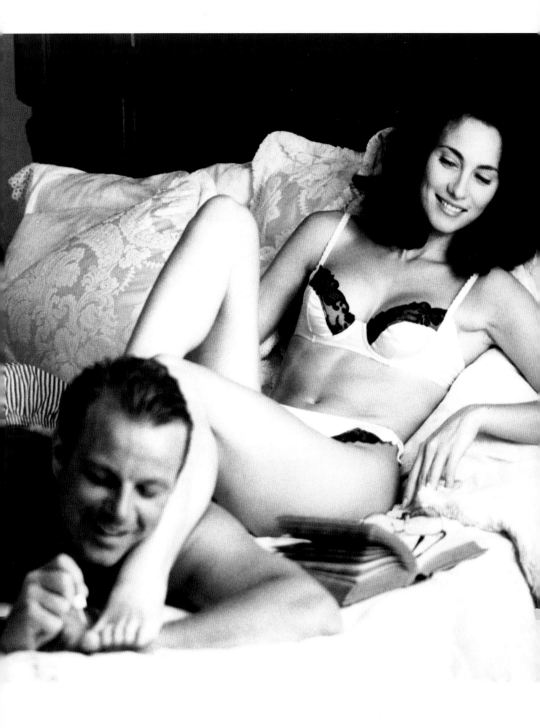

# MODERN POLISH FORMULATIONS

Modern nail polish formulations are now mixed with synthetic resins for maximum gloss, pigment, and wearing properties. They have certainly come a long way from their early formulations.

Today, the basic ingredient in nail lacquer is still nitrocellulose (cellulose nitrate) cotton, a liquid mixed with microscopic cotton fibers. Other ingredients are added: solvents like butyl acetate or ethyl acetate that evaporate quickly, thus speeding up the drying process; film-forming agents; resins and plasticizers; solvents; and coloring agents. Various other resins and plasticizers like castor oil or glycerine are added to improve the flexibility and water resistance of the polish. For polishes with pearlescent finishes, the manufacturers might add mica or even ground-up fish scales.

Nail polish makers have been under pressure to reduce or eliminate potentially toxic ingredients, including phthalates, toluene, and formaldehyde, from their nail polish formulations. There are two ingredients in particular that can cause allergic reactions in sensitive individuals:

### Toluene

is manufactured from petroleum by-products and can cause contact dermatitis; clues to look for might be red and swollen eyelids.

### Formaldehyde

is commonly used in nail hardeners and is a chemical preservative that can cause skin irritation and allergic reactions. The first clue is a rash.

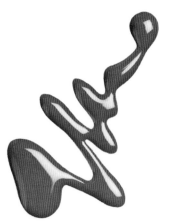

## Allergic reactions

Allergic reactions to nail polish may first appear on your eyelids. If your eyelids become red and swollen after buying a new polish, this is a clue that you may be allergic to some of the ingredients. Because the skin of the eyelids is so delicate, it is particularly susceptible to contact dermatitis, which means your nails or hands have probably rubbed your eyes.

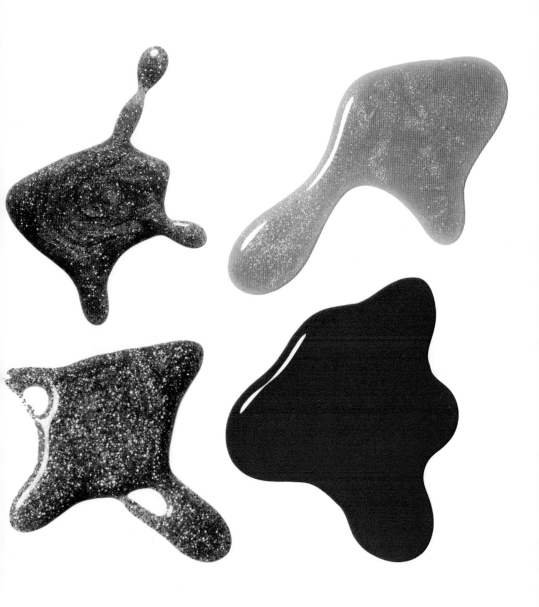

# THE HAND AND FOOT IN DETAIL

Your hands are the main organs for physically manipulating your environment, used for both gross motor skills and fine motor skills. The fingertips contain some of the densest areas of nerve endings on the body, are the richest source of tactile feedback, and have the greatest positioning capability of the body; thus the sense of touch is intimately associated with hands.

Your feet consist of an amazing framework of bones, ligaments, muscles, and tendons, designed to bear the weight of your body efficiently and enable mobility. Each of your feet contains 26 bones, as well as 33 joints, over 100 ligaments, and a complicated network of blood vessels, tendons, and nerves. All of these combined enable you to move fluidly and with balance. The feet also act as the body's shock absorbers and as levers to propel the body forward. The structure of the foot is similar to that of the hand, but the toes lack the mobility of the thumb and fingers.

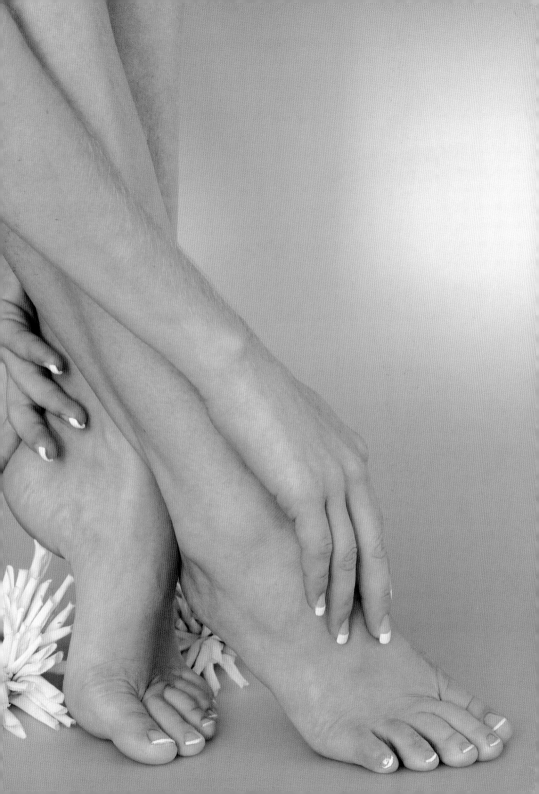

# STRUCTURE

By understanding how they work and knowing how to care for them, you will be able to ensure a lifetime of healthy, strong, and mobile hands and feet.

The skin on the back of the hand, called dorsal skin, is thin and flexible and separate from the underlying tissue—a suppleness essential for the flexibility of the fingers. The skin on the palms of the hands, the soles of the feet, and the gripping surfaces of the fingers and toes is called volar skin, and is thicker and hairless. This skin is also rich in sensory receptors, enabling us to perceive touch, pressure, heat, pain, and surface texture. It is covered with a myriad of rich nerve endings, to enhance sensation; oil glands, to moisturize and waterproof the skin; sweat glands, to excrete toxins and regulate body temperature; and an additional layer, the stratum lucidum, which allows for increased wear and tear. It has more sweat glands to assist in gripping objects and more nerve endings for heightened sensitivity.

Since the hand must be able to flex, the skin needs to be flexible too. Much of this flexibility comes from the arrangement of the deeper tissue over the joints and skin folds. Furrows and creases on the palm and across the back of the hand allow the skin to open and close. These flex folds are located where the skin is connected to deeper tissue, and they permit the hand to close without the skin folding over or bunching.

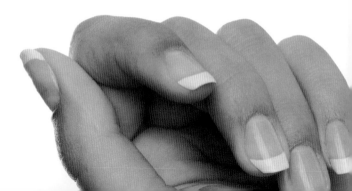

# The skeletal system

### Bones of the arm and hand

Few structures of the human anatomy are as unique or complex as the hand. Mobility, strength, proper alignment, control, and coordination are all essential for normal hand function and all of this is dependent on the structures that make up and move the hand.

There are 64 bones in the arm, wrist, and hand, comprising 10 shoulder and arm bones, 16 wrist, and 38 hand bones.

- The 10 shoulder and arm bones are the clavicle, scapula, humerus, radius, and ulna on each side.
- The 16 wrist bones are the scaphoid, lunate, triquetrum, pisiform, trapezium, trapezoid, capitate, and hamate on each side.
- The 38 hand bones are the 10 metacarpal bones and 28 phalanges.

The humerus is a long bone that extends from the shoulder joint down to the elbow joint. It is weight-bearing and also provides muscle attachment. In the forearm are the ulna and the radius: the ulna is slightly larger than the radius, and runs down the outside of the arm. The two form a joint at the elbow, allowing the lower arm to flex and bend. At the other end, the radius and ulna form a series of joints that connect with the bones of the wrist. There are 27 bones within the wrist and hand. The wrist contains eight small bones, called carpals. The carpals join with the two forearm bones, the

## Did you know?

The function of the hand and wrist is dependent on 27 short bones connected by 30 joints, moved by 34 muscles, which are attached to the bones by tendons from the forearm and hand. Activated by 3 peripheral nerves, these are nourished by a system of arteries, veins, and other support structures.

radius and ulna, forming the wrist joint. In the palm, the main part of the hand, the eight carpal bones connect to the five metacarpal bones that form the palm of the hand. One metacarpal connects to each finger and thumb. Small bone shafts called phalanges line up to form each finger and thumb; there are three of these in each finger, with only two in the thumbs.

### Joints and spaces

A joint is a junction between the ends of two or more bones in the skeleton. A synovial joint is surrounded by the joint capsule, a layer of fibrous tissue, and an inner lining of synovial membrane. This membrane produces a lubricating fluid that nourishes the surfaces of the joints, enabling us to bend, flex, and rotate our fingers, wrists, and elbows.

The main knuckle joints are formed by the connections of the phalanges to the metacarpals. These joints are called the metacarpal phalangeal joints, and work like a hinge when you bend and straighten your fingers and thumb.

The three phalanges in each finger are separated by two joints, called interphalangeal joints. The thumb only has one interphalangeal joint between the two thumb phalanges. All of these interphalangeal joints of the digits also work like a hinge when you bend and straighten your fingers and thumb.

The joints of the hand, fingers, and the thumb are covered at the ends with articular cartilage. This white, shiny material has a rubbery consistency. The function of articular cartilage is to absorb shock and provide an extremely smooth surface to facilitate motion. There is articular cartilage essentially everywhere that two bony surfaces move against one another, or articulate.

Tendons connect the bones of the hand with the bones of the lower arm. This complex framework allows us a full range of fine and gross movement in our fingers, hands, wrists, and arms, adapting to massive tasks as well as the most delicate.

### Bones of the leg and foot

The long bone running down from the thigh is the femur; it extends from the hip to the knee and is

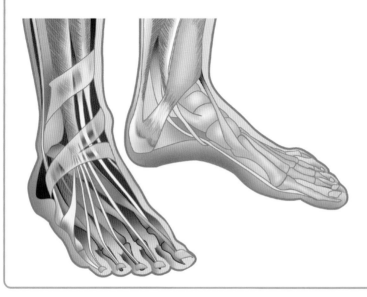

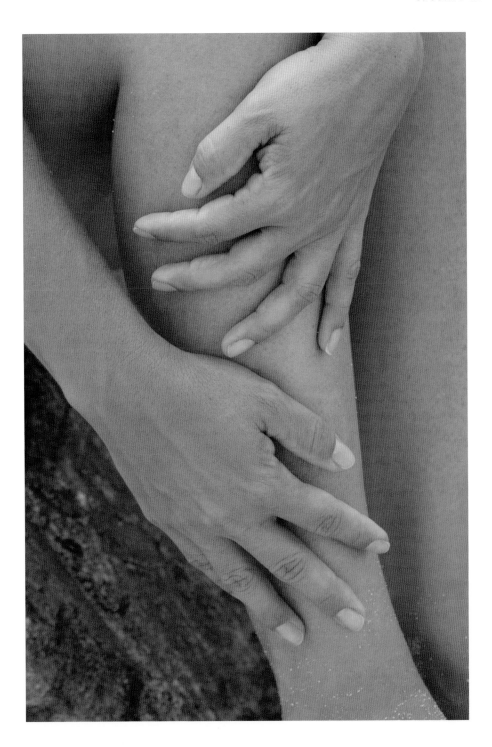

essentially load-bearing. It also provides muscle attachment, and forms a joint at the knee with the bones of the lower leg. The lower leg bones are called the tibia and fibula. The tibia is the long strong bone in the middle of the leg. Its primary function is to support body weight; it forms a joint with the talus at the ankle. The fibula is a long, slim bone situated toward the outer side of the leg and is mainly used for muscle attachment; it forms a joint with the tibia near the knee and extends down to form joints with the ankle. The patella, or kneecap, is a flat bone situated at the knee joint; it forms no joint with any other bones as it is embedded in the tendon of the quadriceps muscle at the front of the thigh.

Your feet are a remarkable framework of bones, ligaments, muscles, and tendons, designed to bear the weight of your body and enable mobility. Together your feet contain 52 bones (a quarter of the bones in your body) as well as 66 joints, over 200 ligaments, and a complex network of blood vessels, tendons, and nerves. Each ankle is made up of seven tarsal bones, which are much larger than the carpals of the hand. They are arranged to support and distribute the body's weight throughout the foot. The calcaneum attaches the lower muscles of the calf to the foot, which enables us to run, walk, and move effectively. On the inside of the talus lies the navicular, which is used for muscle attachment and movement. The five long bones (metatarsals) make up the length of the foot, forming joints with the tarsals at one end and the bones of the foot at the other. The phalanges are arranged in the same way as in the hand; there are 14 in each foot, with two in each toe. Occasionally the phalanges are fused together in the little toes. The heel pad and arches of your foot act as shock absorbers, cushioning the impact and jarring that occur with each and every step. All of this together enables us to move fluidly and with balance—amazingly, the relatively small area of the feet manages to support some 100 to 250 pounds of body weight, acting as levers to propel the body forward when we walk and run. Wear and tear caused by the simplest of chores exerts thousands of tons of pressure onto our feet every day. The average person takes around 8,000 steps each day—so by the time you are in your seventies, you will have covered a distance equivalent to walking around the Earth three times. With all this wear and tear, hard floor surfaces, and poorly designed footwear, it's no wonder so many people have foot problems.

## The muscular system

The muscular system covers, shapes, and supports the skeleton, and is responsible for producing all the movements of the body. The entire muscular system consists of more than 500 muscles, both large and small, which comprise 40 to 50 percent of the weight of the human body. Muscles are fibrous tissues that can stretch and contract according to our movements; different types of movement will depend on muscles performing in specific ways. Muscle movements assist the flow of blood and lymph through the vessels and lymphatic systems. There are three types of muscular tissue:

- Striated, or striped, muscles are voluntary muscles that you can move whenever you want.
- Nonstriated muscles move involuntarily, which means their functioning is automatic (for instance, the stomach and intestine).
- Cardiac, or heart muscle, which is not found anywhere else in the body.

The muscles of the hand don't work alone, but as an interactive group of muscles. There are 20 small muscle groups for independent finger movements, plus an additional 14 muscle groups in the forearm. Nine muscles contribute to the flexibility and strength of the thumb, allowing it greater mobility and range of motion than the other fingers. This is vital, as the thumb needs more strength to oppose the pressure exerted by four fingers.

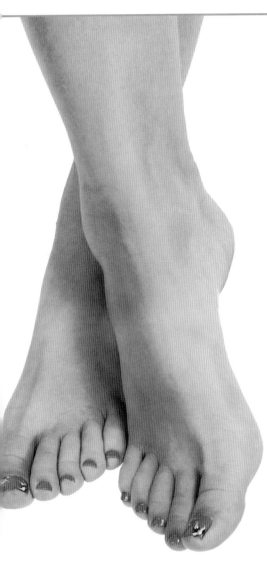

## Ligaments and tendons

Muscles are linked to the bone by thick, inflexible bands of fibrous tissue called tendons. All of the muscle groups are joined to bones by more than 20 long tendons. Ligaments are dense fibrous bands that connect one bone to another, holding them in place but allowing some movement. Tendons connect a muscle to a bone; when the muscle contracts, the strong, cablelike tendon pulls the bone to which it is attached. For instance, the large Achilles tendon links the calf muscle to the heel bone. The tendons enter the hand by passing under a large wristband tendon, and then crisscross around each finger.

## Vascular system

There is a network of fine capillaries carrying blood to maintain the health of the skin. Blood carries nutrients and oxygen to every cell in the body and removes waste products. The blood plays many essential roles in the working of the body:

- It helps regulate body heat by dilating and constricting; if the body becomes cold, the blood vessels will constrict, keeping the blood deeper within the body to conserve heat.
- If the skin is damaged or cut, the blood vessels clot, preventing further blood loss.
- If the body's defense system is triggered by an allergen or irritant, histamine is released, attempting to destroy the invader by increasing blood flow to the area.

**Arteries** carry bright red oxygenated blood, under pressure, away from the heart. They have muscular walls to contain the blood and maintain pressure, which results in the blood moving around the body.

**Veins** carry dark red deoxygenated blood and waste products back to the heart.

**Capillaries** form the link between arteries and veins. They are tiny vessels that thread through the tissues of the body.

# The lymphatic system

A "secondary" system, the lymphatic system, assists the body's blood circulation to rid the body of waste that the veins can't cope with. It plays a vital role in the functioning of the immune system, which is responsible for disease control. The lymphatic system consists of lymph spaces, lymph vessels, and lymph glands.

The lymphatic system starts off as a series of thin-walled tubes or lymphatic vessels. These vessels contain valves, which prevent the back flow of fluid within them. The vessels have a similar structure to the capillaries, although they are more permeable, threading between the cells of the body in much the same way as capillaries do. The lymphatic fluid is filtered by lymph glands situated all over the body. The lymphatic system does not have a pump to move it around, as the blood system does, and is reliant on muscular movement to push it along. Sometimes this flow can be sluggish and excess fluid and waste can build up in certain areas. Fluid not returned to the circulation via the capillaries seeps into the two lymph ducts, where it becomes known as lymph. As the natural movement of the muscles squeezes the ducts, the lymph is forced along them. The lymphatic ducts are joined together by this network of vessels and along their length are lymph nodes, through which the lymph has to pass. These nodes clean the lymph of debris and microbes before it's returned to the general blood circulation.

Lymph fluid is a clear, slightly yellow, watery fluid resembling blood plasma. It contains all the same components as blood plasma except for the plasma proteins, which are lower in concentration. Lymph contains fibrogen, which helps with blood clotting, and leucocytes, which help fight any infection in the body. The tissue found in the tissue spaces bathes all cells and trades its nutritive materials to the cells in return for the water and waste products of metabolism. This fluid is absorbed into the lymphatic or lymph capillaries to become lymph, and is then filtered and detoxified as it passes through the lymph nodes. It is eventually reintroduced into the blood circulation.

Like any waste-removal system, the lymph system works best when the lymph is moving. When it's congested or blocked, waste builds up in the tissue and can cause blemishes, rashes, and irritation on the skin. The way to get the lymph moving is through exercise, walking, dancing, or stretching and, of course, massage. The more efficient the lymph system is at removing toxic substances, the more beautiful your skin becomes. Minimize straining your lymphatic system by avoiding excess consumption of artificial substances, alcohol, animal fats, cholesterol, and smoking.

The primary functions of the lymphatic system are as follows:
- To drain tissue fluid from all organs.
- To remove waste material from the body cells to the blood.
- To carry nourishment from the blood to the body cells.
- To act as a bodily defense against invading bacteria and toxins.
- To reach the parts of the body not reached by blood and to carry on an interchange with the blood.
- To prevent the waterlogging of tissues.
- To transport fats from the small intestine, or ileum, to the liver.
- To produce fibrogen.
- To produce lymphocytes.
- To return protein molecules to the blood, which are unable to pass back through the capillary walls due to their size.
- To prevent edema, the excessive swelling of fluid in the tissues, which leads to localized swelling, usually due to standing for long periods, or to an obstruction in the lymph drainage pathway, such as an infected lymph node.

# The nervous system

Three main nerves in the hand allow you to feel sensation, experience motion, and participate in fine, delicate movement. The median nerve is the main nerve for precision grip; it controls the finger and wrist flexion. It also controls sensation in the palm-side surface of the thumb, index, and middle fingers and half of the ring finger, as well as supplying stimulus to the muscles that bring the thumb toward the fingers to enable you to grasp an object. The ulnar nerve works with the median to innervate the muscles responsible for the fine motor movements of the hand, affecting the muscles that extend the arm, forearm, hand, and fingers.

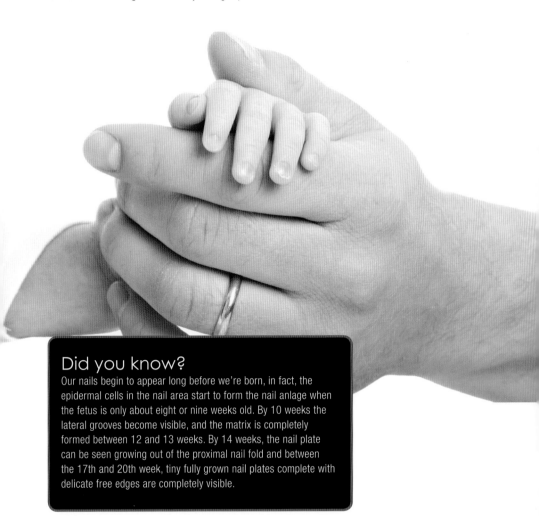

## Did you know?

Our nails begin to appear long before we're born, in fact, the epidermal cells in the nail area start to form the nail anlage when the fetus is only about eight or nine weeks old. By 10 weeks the lateral grooves become visible, and the matrix is completely formed between 12 and 13 weeks. By 14 weeks, the nail plate can be seen growing out of the proximal nail fold and between the 17th and 20th week, tiny fully grown nail plates complete with delicate free edges are completely visible.

# THE SKIN

A waterproof yet washable, flexible material that can mend and repair itself—your skin is the perfect protective shield.

The body's outer covering, your skin, is the first line of defense against the environment, protecting us against damage from heat and light, and from injury and infection. It regulates body temperature; eliminates toxins; stores water, fat, and vitamin D; and warms and cools us. The single largest organ of the body, it covers between 14 and 21 square feet and weighs around 7 pounds, depending on your size.

The skin has eight main functions: protection, storage, excretion, sensation, secretion, vitamin D formation, absorption, and temperature regulation.

**1 Protection** The skin provides a waterproof covering that protects against bacterial infections, dirt, chemical attack, and minor injuries. Its initial barrier of oil (sebum) and sweat forms an acidic film, discouraging bacterial and fungal growth and helping prevent the skin losing and absorbing too much water. Finally, melanin protects against ultraviolet rays.

**2 Storage** The skin serves as an emergency reservoir for fat and water.

**3 Excretion** Perspiration and some waste products like water and salt are lost through the skin.

**4 Sensation** Different nerve endings in the skin respond to heat, cold, pressure, touch, and pain.

**5 Secretion** Sebum, which moisturizes and protects, is secreted from the sebaceous glands.

**6 Vitamin D formation** Vitamin D is produced via ultraviolet (UV) rays, which are essential for the absorption of calcium.

**7 Absorption** Although fairly limited, some substances can be absorbed though the skin, like antibiotics, aromatherapy oils, and certain chemicals.

**8 Heat regulation** Dilation or constriction of the blood vessels (capillaries) regulates the body's temperature; sweat produced by the sweat glands cools and evaporates; and fat in the subcutaneous layer insulates the body.

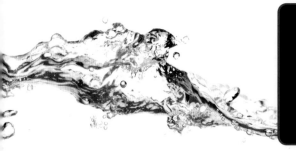

## Did you know?

An area of 0.15 inches squared contains: 9.7 feet of blood vessels, 200 nerve endings, 38.6 feet of nerves, 15 sebaceous glands, 100 sudiferous glands, and approximately 10 hairs.

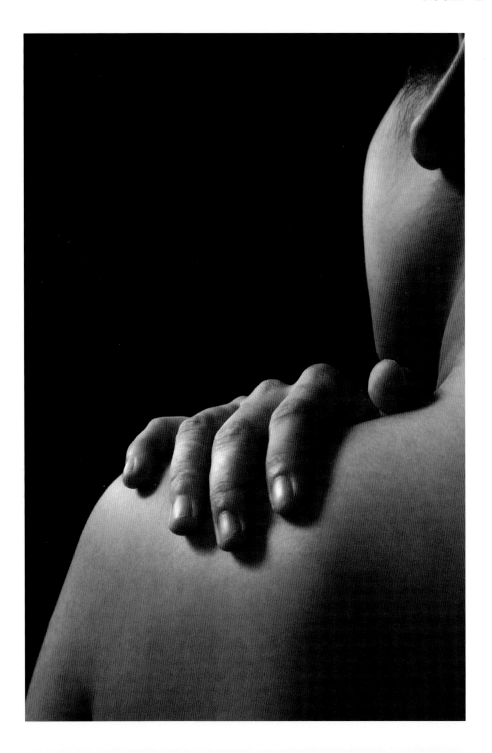

# The layers of the skin

The skin is made up of three main layers: the epidermis (outer layer), the dermis (inner layer), and the subcutaneous layer.

## The epidermis

The epidermis (outer layer), or top, translucent layer, is entirely protective in function. It is responsible for protection from bacterial and fungal growth, UV rays, and mechanical damage, and for the entry and exit of substances like water and chemicals. This self-repairing, self-renewing layer lies just below the stratum corneum, averaging 0.002 inches (0.07 mm). It is made up of scalelike cells composed of keratin, and flat, scalelike squamous cells. Below these are the round basal cells. The deepest part of the epidermis also contains melanocytes, which produce melanin, which give the skin its color. The epidermal layer consists mainly of keratinocytes—in various stages of growth, maturation, and death—and makes up five layers—stratum basale, stratum spinosum, stratum granulosum, stratum luciderm, and stratum corneum.

## The dermis

This inner layer of skin is composed of connective tissue, which is embedded with blood vessels, lymph ducts, sensory nerve endings, blood capillaries, sweat, and sebaceous glands, hair follicles, and follicle muscles. It carries a vast network of capillaries and gives structural support. The dermis is responsible for most sensory and glandular functioning of the skin, the nutrition of the area, and excretion and secretion within the skin, and it assists temperature control. Glands produce sweat, which helps regulate body temperature, and sebum, an oily substance that helps keep the skin from drying out. Sweat and sebum reach the skin's surface through tiny openings called pores. One of the main features of the dermis is the network of strong collagen and elastin fibers. Collagen acts as a support to the skin and keeps it plump and youthful, while elastin allows the skin to stretch, move, and return to its original position. In young skin these fibers are plentiful, but as the skin ages they break down and the lack of collagen allows the formation of wrinkles between the muscles. Diminished elastin becomes more evident as the skin becomes softer and less firm.

## The subcutaneous layer

Beneath these two layers is the subcutaneous, adipose, or fatty layer, made up of fatty tissue also known as adipose tissue, which is responsible for heat insulation, energy storage, and cushioning. Attached to the dermis by connective tissue, it serves as a protective cushion for the muscles and bone. Situated beneath the dermis layer, containing large blood vessels and primarily fat-filled cells called adipose cells, it also contains a network of arteries that run parallel to the surface subcutaneous layer, branching into smaller capillary networks around hair follicles, sebaceous and sweat glands, and lymph.

## Did you know?

- Your skin makes up about 16% of your total body weight.
- Your skin sheds 30,000 to 40,000 dead skin cells almost every minute.
- Your skin renews itself every 28 days.
- Your skin swells when it absorbs water.

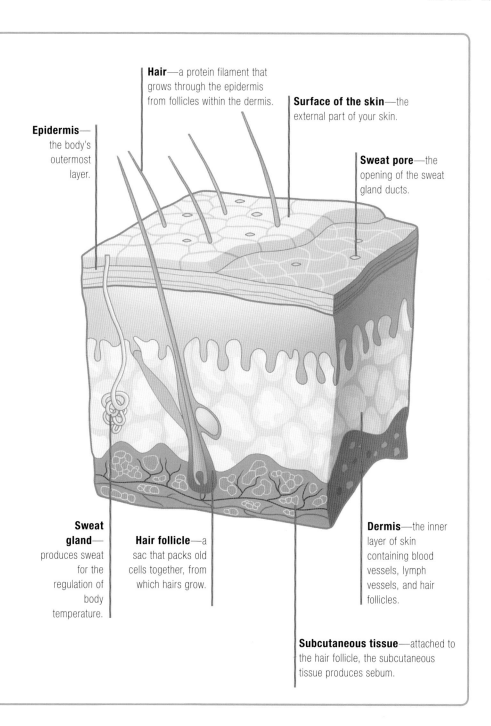

**Hair**—a protein filament that grows through the epidermis from follicles within the dermis.

**Surface of the skin**—the external part of your skin.

**Epidermis**—the body's outermost layer.

**Sweat pore**—the opening of the sweat gland ducts.

**Sweat gland**—produces sweat for the regulation of body temperature.

**Hair follicle**—a sac that packs old cells together, from which hairs grow.

**Dermis**—the inner layer of skin containing blood vessels, lymph vessels, and hair follicles.

**Subcutaneous tissue**—attached to the hair follicle, the subcutaneous tissue produces sebum.

# Skin problems

### ◕ Contact dermatitis (eczema)

Contact dermatitis is an allergic reaction to certain substances touching the skin. Symptoms include itching, redness, and dryness. When it affects nails and the surrounding skin, irritants like adhesives, monomers, or primers used to secure acrylic nails are probably the cause. Stop using the irritating substance or consult a dermatologist if you are unsure of the cause. Often confused with psoriasis or onychomycosis, an infectious disease caused by fungus, it results in white patches that can be scraped off the nail, or yellowish streaks within the nail.

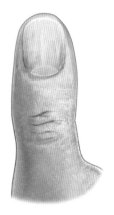

### Allergic reactions

A swelling, rash, open sore, or inflammation may be an indication of an allergic reaction to a particular product or chemical. In some cases, the nail may become white in color or have white patches. When the skin is inflamed or irritated by a foreign substance, the immune system will react. The area becomes swollen and the blood releases histamines, which enlarge the vessels around the injury, enabling blood to rush quickly to the affected area and help remove the irritation. If you are prone to allergic reactions, it would be a good idea to carry out a skin test on a nail; if in doubt, consult a dermatologist.

### Fungal or yeast infections

Can often invade the superficial layers of the skin, resulting in infection. Usually germinating their spores alongside the edges of fingernails and toenails, some fungal infections are caused by microscopic plantlike organisms related to mushrooms and yeast, invading through a tear in the nail fold. These are normally white or yellowish in color and may affect the texture and shape of the nails as the fungus eats away at the keratin protein of the nail plate. As the infection develops, the nail may darken and discolor, becoming thickened and crumbly. Poor hygiene can cause fungus to develop. Sterilize the tools in your nail kit with an antibacterial spray. The first problem is getting it diagnosed accurately; if a fungus problem persists, it is best to consult a dermatologist. Relatively rare on fingernails, they are most often found on toenails. Fungi prefer dark, warm, and moist areas; feet and shoes provide an ideal breeding ground.

### Herpes simplex (cold sores)

A highly contagious viral infection, usually seen around the mouth; care must be taken to prevent cross-infection.

### Psoriasis

Usually presents as round, reddish, dry spots and patches covered with silvery scales. When it affects the nail plate, the nail becomes pitted and dry, may change color, and separates from the nail bed. If severe, the nail plate may disintegrate completely. It's best to consult a dermatologist if evidence of psoriasis is visible.

### Tinea pedis (athlete's foot)

The most common type of skin infection of the feet. It is a fungal infection that often occurs on the bottom of the feet, but it is usually found on the webs between the toes and can spread to other parts of the foot. Most common forms of this infection include the "moccasin form" and the interdigital form. The moccasin form gets its name from the fact that it covers the entire bottom surface of the foot; in severe cases the foot may have small, scaly rings. Feet with the interdigital form are scaly and itchy with skin that splits between the toes. It often has a reddish border extending beyond the white scales; the red area increases in size as the infection spreads. Chronic infections can last for over six months and can be controlled, although not always cured. Over-the-counter antifungal medication is available and is very effective, so taking oral prescription medication may be unnecessary. Exfoliating helps to improve the skin condition. It is safe to pedicure feet with mild athlete's foot or other mild fungal infections, provided normal salon hygiene practices are followed and all implements are sanitized and disinfected.

### Tinea unguium (ringworm of the nails)

A rare condition that will affect more than one nail if it occurs. The affected area turns gray or yellow and the nails become very brittle. In some cases, the nail plate may separate from the nail bed. If the nail has been affected, the main symptoms are red lesions occurring in patches or rings. Itching may be slight or severe and treatment would be the same for both hands and feet. This condition is highly contagious and contraindicates all treatments—a doctor will need to be consulted.

### Impetigo

Impetigo is an extremely contagious skin disease, usually caused by the bacteria staphylococcus. It starts with the formation of vesicles on the skin, which later dry up, leaving yellow-brown scabs, the discharge from which is highly contagious. Primarily found on the face, the disease spreads easily to other areas of the skin.

### Scabies

Scabies appears as a raised itchy rash and is caused by a mite. It is highly contagious and transmitted by direct contact. It contraindicates all treatments, so refer yourself to a doctor if you suspect you may have symptoms.

### ⬇ Warts

Raised lumps of horny tissue caused by a highly contagious viral infection. Untreatable and must be referred to a doctor.

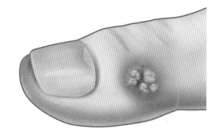

## Did you know?

Doctors often use the condition of the nails to diagnose physical problems.

# THE STRUCTURE AND COMPOSITION OF THE NATURAL NAIL

Nails serve many purposes, but their primary function is to protect and shield the delicate nerve endings and the soft skin at the tips of our fingers, as well as provide support to the soft tissues of the fingers and toes. They also help to enhance the fingertips' sensation, which improves precision and increases the sensation of touch.

## Nail structure

Nails aid dexterity, are useful when picking things up, and enable you to scratch, grasp, and even pinch. Like hair, they are made up of a fibrous protein called keratin, which gives the nails their protective, hard quality. Nails vary in thickness from around 0.02 inches (0.5mm) to 0.03 inches (0.75mm) and are usually convex in shape. The nail's coloration is a delicate shade of pink due to the network of blood vessels beneath them; sometimes they appear lighter when it's cold and the blood vessels have constricted. This semitransparent, flattish, and mostly rectangular plate is made up of several components, but their main component is keratin—a tough fibrous protein polymer made from amino acids and thought to be about 100 cells thick. The structure of the nail can be divided into three main regions—the root, the body, and the border—or six specific parts—the root, nail bed, nail plate, eponychium (cuticle), perionychium, and hyponychium. Each of these structures has a specific purpose, and if disrupted or interfered with in any way, can result in an abnormal-appearing fingernail.

### Nail matrix (root)

Nail growth begins in the nail matrix, or root; it is the living part of the nail hidden underneath the eponychium. The root of the nail rests on and grows from a thick area of epidermal cells known as the germinal matrix, which is not actually visible, and lies underneath a curved fold of epidermis (the proximal nail fold or mantle). It extends several millimeters into the finger and is closely bound by fibrous tissue to the tip surface of the underlying phalangeal bone. "Proximal" is the medical term meaning "nearest"; in this case, referring to the fold nearest the point where the nail attaches. This is the area where the cells divide and produce keratinocytes (the cells that make up keratin). As more and more nail cells are produced, the older ones are pushed outward and flattened, resulting in the cells becoming transparent and part of the nail plate, losing their original white, plump appearance. The developing nail within the matrix is very soft until full keratinization has taken place. Any severe bangs or damage in this area can result in a permanently deformed nail. The shape of the matrix will determine the thickness and width of the nail—the longer the matrix, the thicker the nail—while the shape of the fingertip bone determines whether the nail plate is flat, ski-jump, arched, or hooked.

## The nail bed and nail plate

The most evident part of the nail is the nail plate, a hard, smooth, slightly convex covering; this lies upon the appropriately named nail bed, which is the bed of tissue. The nail plate extends from the edge of the germinal matrix, or lunula, to the hyponychium, and contains the blood vessels, nerves, and melanocytes, or melanin-producing cells, which nourish the nail.

As keratin forms in the nail matrix, it pushes forward onto the nail bed, hardening and becoming the translucent nail plate, or the actual fingernail. The nail plate acts as a protective shield and is composed of carbon, oxygen, nitrogen, hydrogen, sulfur, and trace elements of calcium, magnesium, manganese, zinc, iron, and copper. The underside of the nail plate has grooves along the length of the nail that help anchor it to the nail bed. As we age, the nail plate becomes thinner and vertical ridges start to appear.

## The eponychium

The skin that lies directly on top of the newly developed nail plate is called the eponychium; its function is to act as a barrier seal to prevent bacteria and possible infection entering the matrix.

Often incorrectly referred to as the cuticle, the cuticle is, in fact, only a part of the eponychium, found on the underside of the eponychium where the tissue sits against the newly forming nail plate. This tissue sticks to the freshly made nail, and it's this thin layer of dead tissue that is the cuticle. During a manicure, the

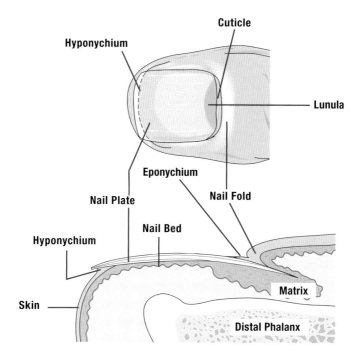

eponychium is gently pushed back to expose the cuticle. The eponychium attaches closely to the nail plate and moves with it as the nail plate grows. This extra growth of eponychium is generally freed and pushed back during a manicure. This important part of the seal protects the nail matrix; if treated too aggressively or handled too roughly, the matrix seal can be broken and infection can occur.

## Perionychium

The sides of the nail are lined with a curved fold of skin known as the lateral fold or wall. The cornified layer of nail extends fractionally onto the nail plate, forming another protective seal. The perionychium is usually where we find hangnails, ingrown nails, and an infection of the skin called paronychia.

## Hyponychium

The hyponychium is the area of skin at the end of the nail bed between the "free edge" of the nail and the skin of the fingertip. It provides a waterproof barrier, or seal, and prevents bacteria, fungi, and viruses from attacking the nail bed. Made up of epidermal tissue, it is a thin strip of tissue that attaches the two lateral nail folds. The epidermal cells here are constantly being shed and sometimes a build up can be found under the free edge, especially of the toenail where they get trapped. With many nerve endings, which act as a warning to this seal being broken, any damage to this area can result in serious infection that could result in the loss of the nail plate.

## The nail folds

The nail folds protect the matrix; both the proximinal (nearest attached end) nail fold and the lateral nail folds are part of our skin. The skin does not just end there; in fact, it folds at the edges and continues underneath, acting as a protective barrier, sealing and protecting the matrix against bacteria and dirt. The lateral nail fold is an extension of the proximal nail fold and protects each side of the nail plate.

## The onychodermal band

This is the area between the nail plate and the hyponychium. It can be recognized by a slight change of color. When applying a French manicure, it is referred to as the "smile line" and it should, ideally, mirror the shape of the base of the nail.

## The lunula

Often referred to as the half-moon or the visible part of the matrix. The whitish half-moons are keratin cells that have not yet been completely flattened or fully keratinized. The lunula is normally more prominent on the thumbs. The area over the lunula is the thinnest part of the nail plate and the easiest to damage or puncture, especially with sharp implements. Any injury or damage to this area can result in permanent nail damage.

# Nail growth

Nails grow all the time, but the rate of growth differs from person to person, and from finger to finger. Fast-growing nails indicate good health, while slower growth can be attributed to illness, poor circulation, some medications, or inadequate diet. Fingernails will inevitably grow faster than toenails, at a rate of around 0.1 inches (3mm) per month, taking around six months for a nail to grow all the way from the matrix to the free edge. It takes five to six months to completely replace the entire nail plate and one to two months for a new nail plate to grow out from the matrix to just past the eponychium. Toenails grow at a much slower rate, about 0.04 inches (1 mm) per month, and can take 12–18 months to be completely replaced.

Your age, the state of your health, a well-balanced diet, and even the weather, all play a contributing role in how fast your nails grow. Growing faster in our early years, our nails reach their growth peak in puberty and gradually slow down as we get older. Growth is accelerated in the summer, during pregnancy, and when we sleep. Each nail grows at a different rate, with our "pinkies," and then the thumbs, being the slowest, and the index finger generally growing much faster than the other fingers.

Trauma and impact can seriously affect the nail plate; any damage to the matrix will affect the growth pattern, and can even result in permanent deformity. Chemical damage can occur when using hazardous materials without protecting your nails.

Water can also be very destructive, especially when hands are constantly exposed to it without protection—so take heed. Rubber gloves are essential when submerging your hands for long periods of time.

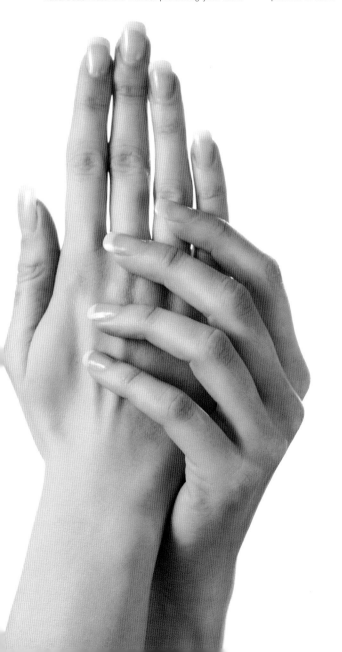

# Fingertip facts—Did you know?

- Fingernails reflect your state of health. Brittle, pale, or bluish fingernails can indicate problems such as thyroid, anemia, vitamin or mineral deficiencies, and liver trouble. Horizontal ridges or small indentations can indicate high stress in your recent past.

- Nails that are naturally thick or thin are hereditary; it all depends on the shape of the matrix.

- Other than the palmar interossei (small muscles in the hand that lie on the anterior of the metacarpals) fingers don't have muscles. Fingers are actually moved by tendons, which are moved by the muscles of the forearm.

- Most autistic children don't point; this is used as a diagnostic test for autism.

- Men often have longer ring fingers than index fingers; this is caused by differences in estrogen and testosterone levels.

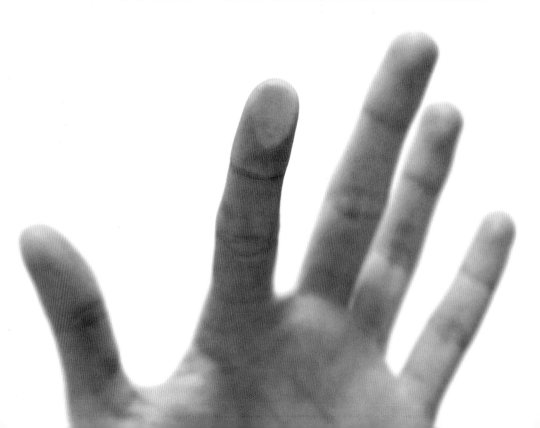

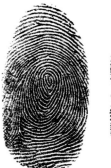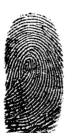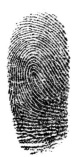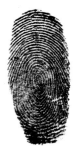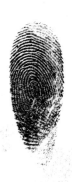

- Fingers are never perfectly straight. Usually, the index, ring, and small finger curve slightly sideways toward the middle finger, and the middle finger may curve toward either side.

- Aside from the genitals, the fingertips possess the highest concentration of touch receptors in all areas of the skin, making them extremely sensitive to heat, cold, pressure, vibration, texture, and moisture.

- The muscles that power the fingers are very strong; strong enough to climb vertical surfaces and support their entire weight at times by just a few fingertips. The biomechanics of the hand require that the force generated by the muscles, which bend the fingertips, must be at least four times the pressure produced at the fingertips.

- The thumb is controlled by nine individual muscles, which are controlled by all three major hand nerves.

- The expression, "If you can move your finger, it isn't broken," is false.

- There is no evidence to support the statement, "Eating gelatin makes your fingernails stronger."

- About one in ten people are left-handed.

- Only about two in one hundred people are ambidextrous.

- No two people have identical fingerprints.

# NAIL DISEASES AND DISORDERS

A thorough understanding of the conditions that can affect the nail will help you learn to recognize nails that are infected, deformed, or otherwise unhealthy or simply neglected. This will enable you to keep your nails in peak condition. Nail conditions that show signs of infection or inflammation require medical assistance.

**Anonychia** Anonychia (absence of nails) is a rare congenital condition.

**Bruised nails** Usually caused by a clot of blood forming under the nail after impact or trauma. Sometimes the nail plate can be pierced to relieve pressure, but this will need to be done by a professional.

**Beau's lines** Horizontal, traversing ridges on the nail, usually caused by illness.

⊕ **Brittle nails** Tend to have low water content, which will affect the flexibility of the nails. Nail varnishes and oils help prevent loss of water and encourage flexibility.

**Eggshell nails** Thin and very curved on the free edge, often dipping in the center and with a white free edge. Avoid wet manicures, as the nail plate will absorb the water and change shape, straightening when the nail dries and resulting in the polish flaking off.

⊕ **Furrows** Either run horizontally, lengthwise, or vertically across the nail plate. Lengthwise ridges are normal and increase with age, whereas ridges that run across the nail are usually caused by illness, trauma, or poor circulation.

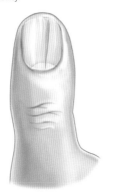

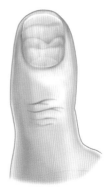

**⊕ Hangnails** Caused by dry cuticles or often resulting from cuticles being cut. Oils and regular manicures can help solve this problem.

**⊕ Leukonychia** White spots or discoloration appears on the nail plate; usually caused by accidental bruising or trauma to the nail matrix.

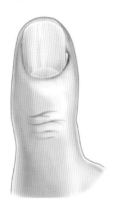

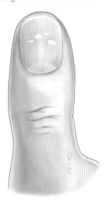

**Hapalonychia** Also known as eggshell nails—a thinning of the fingernails, and/or toenails, that results in the free edge of the nail breaking or bending, with cracks that run lengthwise.

**⊕ Hematoma** A clot of blood, or bruise, forms between the nail plate and the nail bed, usually caused by trauma.

**Melanonychia** Also known as *Melanonchia Striata*, vertical pigmented brown or black stripes form in the nail matrix. Could indicate malignant melanoma or lesions that require medical advice.

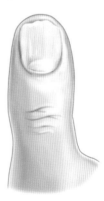

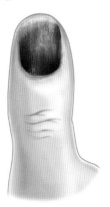

**⊕ Mold** A fungal infection of the nail, usually caused by moisture seeping between artificial nail and free edge of the nail.

**Koilonychia** Literally means "spoon-shaped nails" and refers to nails that flatten, lose their convex contour, and are replaced by a central concave contour with raised edges that loses its natural color. The nail usually becomes thin and brittle.

**Onychatrophia** Atrophying, or wasting away, of the nail plate, which loses shine, shrinks, and sometimes falls off. Can be caused by injury, disease, or nutritional and hereditary conditions.

**Onychauxis or hypertrophy** Thickened nails caused by old age, psoriasis, trauma, etc. Usually caused by internal imbalances, local infection, and in some cases, hereditary factors.

**Onychia** Infection in or on the nail plate, either post-traumatic or with paronychia, often caused by unsanitized manicuring implements. Redness, soreness, or pus is also evident.

**Onychoclasis** Refers to a broken nail, normally occurring at the free edge.

⊕ **Onychogryphosis** The nail plate becomes thick and clawlike. If the nail is not kept short, the curvature can make the nail look like a ram's horn when it extends over the tip of the nail; usually hereditary or the result of psoriasis or trauma.

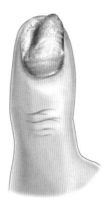

**Onycholysis** Nail separation or loosening from the nail bed usually caused by trauma to the free edge, psoriasis, or an allergic reaction to nail products or drugs.

**Onychomadesis** Nail shedding usually caused by mechanical trauma to the natural nail.

**Onychomycosis** Fungal infection of the nail and probably the most common disease of the nails. Causes fingernails and toenails to thicken, discolor, disfigure, and split. Onychomycosis is caused by dermatophytes (fungi that infect hair, skin, and nails) and feed on keratinized (nail) tissue; also known as tinea unguium (tinea of the nails). This is initially a cosmetic concern. However, if left untreated, the nails become so thickened that they press against the inside of the shoes, causing pressure, discomfort, and pain. Consult a podiatrist or dermatologist.

**Onychophagy** The medical term for nails that have been bitten enough to become deformed. Some biters tear or bite the skin around the nail or the cuticles and sidewalls; others bite the free edge. Nail extensions can help discourage nail-biting, but if the skin is broken or infected, they will only exacerbate the problem.

**Onychophyma** Swelling or hypertrophy of the nails.

**Onychorrhexis** Also known as "brittle nails," this is a brittleness that occurs, meaning the nails tend to split or break, usually splitting lengthwise. Can be caused by mechanical trauma, excessive soap and water exposure, nail polish remover, anorexia or bulimia, and in some cases the overuse of chemical solvents.

**Onychosis** A condition of atrophy or dystrophy of the nails, usually caused by a dermatosis such as a fungal infection.

**Onychotillomania** The habit of deliberate self-inflicted damage done by habitually picking or compulsive manipulation of the nails, causing dystrophy of the nail plate as it grows.

**⊕ Paronychia** A chronic infectious bacterial or fungal infection where inflammation of the tissue around the nail results in redness and tenderness, usually where the nail and skin meet at the side or base of a fingernail or toenail. Usually treated with antibiotics.

**⊕ Psoriasis** An inherited skin condition characterized by silvery shiny scales and round reddish spots. When it affects the nail plate, the nail becomes pitted and dry, thickening abnormally, and possibly disintegrating altogether. Consult a dermatologist.

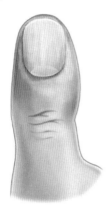

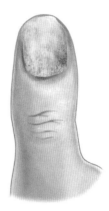

**Pterygium** Abnormal growth of the cuticle over the nail plate, usually caused by trauma to the matrix. Nail loss is usually inevitable.

**⊕ Pseudomonas** A bacterial infection that occurs between the natural nail plate and the nail bed. Thrives in dark spaces, feeds off dead tissue; the darker the discoloration, the worse the infection.

## Pro Tip

To keep fingernails healthy and strong, eat a healthy diet, including vitamins and mineral-rich food. Key vitamins for the nails are vitamins A, B-complex, C, D, E, iron, calcium, magnesium, zinc, sulfur, and essential fatty acids (EFA). But remember, these elements taken as supplements will be ineffectual unless combined with a healthy diet. Nails grow slowly so it will take three to four months before any improvement becomes evident. Creams, oils, and lotions, on the other hand, are sometimes sold as "growth accelerators"; these claims are misleading, as the only effect these products have is beautifying and moisturizing the nail plate.

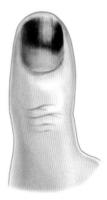

**Trachyonychia** A condition characterized by roughness on the surface of the nail plate, often associated with eczema, psoriasis, and alopecia areata.

# Chapter 2

# EQUIPMENT AND TOOLS

The setting up of equipment and tools can be quite daunting, as the list is seemingly very long. Research and experience will guide you through your choices; look at Internet sites, trade magazines, and trade shows to get a complete overview of the industry and to decide which equipment will apply to you. Not everyone is skilled enough to airbrush, for instance, so you might not need to go to the expense of purchasing an airbrush. Specialized equipment is listed under those specific sections where it is used.

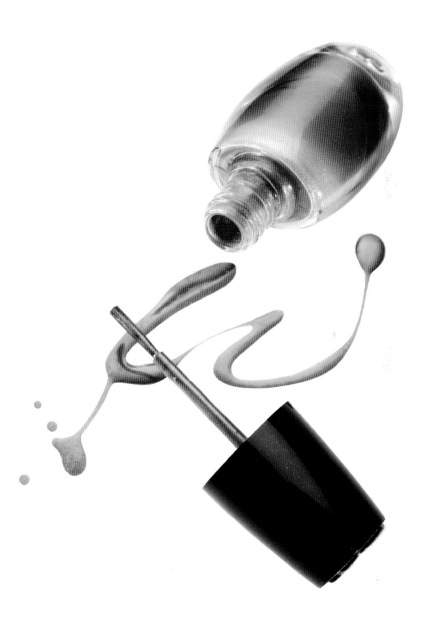

# GEARING UP

The following items will be needed in addition to the standard manicure tools.

## Equipment

- A well-lit and ventilated work surface is essential, preferably with some drawers to contain equipment and keep the work surface uncluttered. Ventilation is crucial, as the dust and fumes created in these treatments is harmful in the long-term; care must be taken to prevent excessive inhalation.
- Desk lamp—bright direct light is crucial for accuracy and neatness, to avoid eye strain while carrying out close work, for checking artificial nail imperfections, and for applying polish and nail art.
- Protective eyewear—should be worn when clipping back tips to protect against flying particles.
- A UV light-source lamp that often looks like a little oven—used to set the gels if UV gel nail extensions are being applied.
- Waste bin—should ideally be a covered metal flip-top.
- Towels—which you can cover with disposable paper towels to help cut down on laundry.
- Manicure bowl—ideally glass or ceramic for dissolving products with which to remove nail tips and acrylic overlays, and for holding warm soapy water to soak fingers during the process.
- Pedicure bowl or foot spa—some technicians like the electric spa bath, but a simple bowl filled with soapy water is more than adequate.
- Glass dappen dishes—initially developed for mixing dental fillings, these are used to store small quantities of monomer when applying enhancements; being small, they help reduce the amount of evaporation.
- Magnifying glass—for close inspection of possible infections or nail conditions.
- Glass jar—for containing antiseptic solution or surgical spirits to sterilize implements.

## Disposables

- Antibacterial soap—ideally stored in a pump applicator, can be used to sanitize your hands. You may prefer using a sanitizing gel or spray.
- Cotton balls or cotton wipes—used to remove nail enamel and to wrap around the end of an orange stick. You may prefer fiber-free squares to remove polish, as they don't leave tiny cotton fibers on the nails that could ruin your nail polish application.
- Lint-free pads—essential for removal of nail polish. They have a slight abrasive quality that eases removal of product and they don't leave fibers behind to spoil your polish application.
- Orangewood stick—ideal for loosening the cuticle and cleaning under the free edge. Made out of orange wood, which doesn't splinter and is nonabsorbent.
- Paper towel—useful for covering cotton towels, preventing nail polish stains, and collecting filing residue.

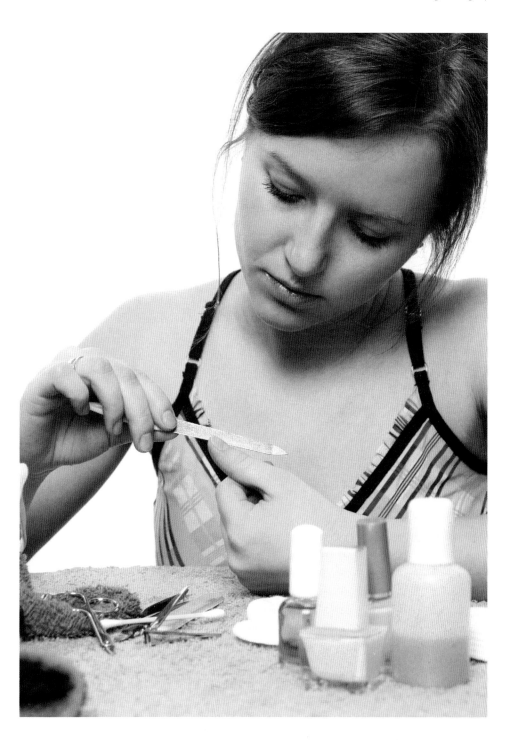

# Tools and implements

- Brushes (for acrylics and gels)—look for good-
  quality sable brushes for durability; they say a
  craftsman is as good as his tools, so take heed.

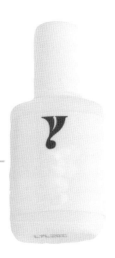

**Brush on nail glue** Essential
for attaching tips.

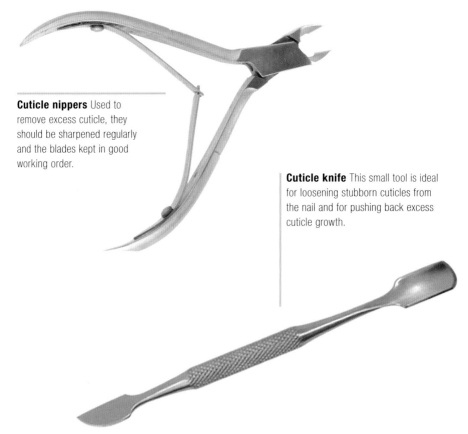

**Cuticle nippers** Used to
remove excess cuticle, they
should be sharpened regularly
and the blades kept in good
working order.

**Cuticle knife** This small tool is ideal
for loosening stubborn cuticles from
the nail and for pushing back excess
cuticle growth.

**Emery board and files** Usually double-sided, one side is coarsely grained and used to shape the nail. The other, fine-grained, side is ideal for beveling the nail or smoothing the free edge.

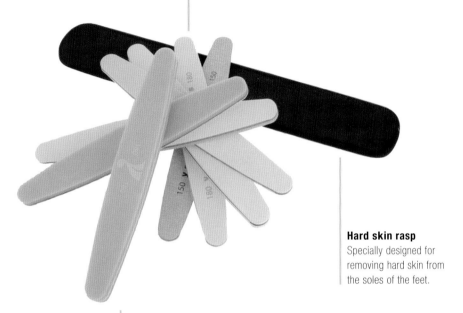

**Hard skin rasp**
Specially designed for removing hard skin from the soles of the feet.

**Magic wand** This wacky tool serves many purposes: One end is a C-curve tool and reverse pincher, while the other is a pusher and scraper. Use the spoon end to push back a cuticle, then turn over to scrape away protein buildup. Use the reverse pincher to hold a nail tip in place after gluing, or use the pincher to create the perfect C-curve.

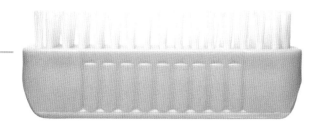

**Nail brush** Essential for cleaning fingernails and toenails and removing debris and grease.

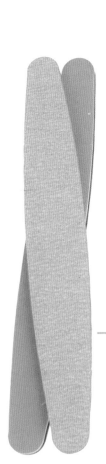

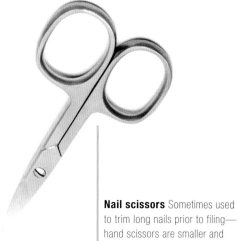

**Nail scissors** Sometimes used to trim long nails prior to filing—hand scissors are smaller and curved, while toe scissors are a lot sturdier with shorter, thicker blades and longer, sprung handles to provide more control.

**Nail buffers** Available in all shapes and sizes, buffers usually combine three different grades of buffing surfaces and help smooth out any ridges on the nail surfaces, as well as adding a sheen. The original bufferx was the chamois buffer, but newer, plasticized versions are also used.

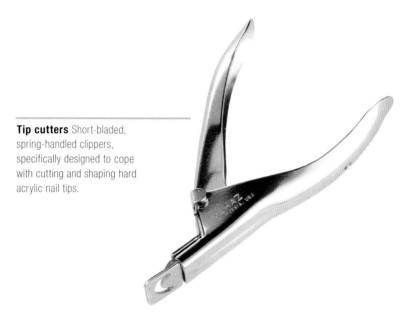

**Tip cutters** Short-bladed, spring-handled clippers, specifically designed to cope with cutting and shaping hard acrylic nail tips.

**Toenail clippers** For cutting flat toe and fingernails. Curved nails may shatter if clipped, so always clip the nail in two parts after it is pre-soaked in warm water to soften and reduce the chance of breakage.

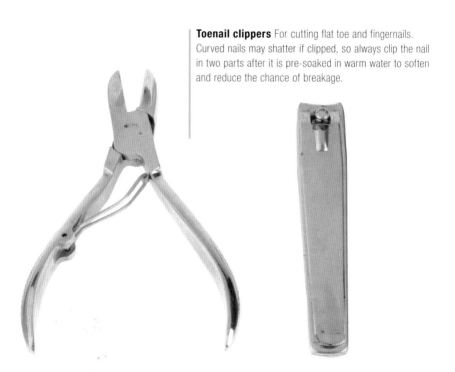

# MATERIALS AND PRODUCTS

Having all your equipment, materials, and products to hand before you start is crucial. Whatever brand you decide to go with, here is a basic guideline of what you'll need.

1 **Soak** Disinfects and cleanses the hands or feet prior to treatment.

2 **Manicure bowl** Holds soapy water in which to soak your fingers. For removal of acrylic nails, float a smaller bowl of acetone in a bowl of hot water to assist in speeding up the removal process.

3 **Acetone-free polish remover** Won't damage or disintegrate nail extensions.

4 **Sanitizer** Sprayed onto hands and feet prior to beginning the manicure process. Cleanses and helps prevent the spread of bacteria and germs. Triclosan and SD alcohol sterilize and help kill bacteria while aloe vera softens and conditions.

5 **Cotton wipes** For removing nail polish and degreasing the nail prior to polish application.

6 **Hand cream or lotion** Softens and smoothes the hands, helping the skin retain moisture.

7 **Soap-free cleanser** Helps hands feel silky smooth. Doesn't leave a residue on nails or interfere with the adherence of base coats and polish.

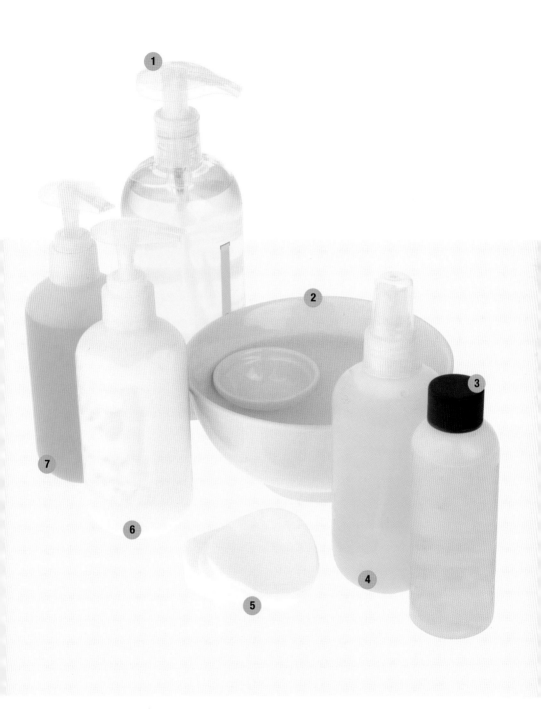

1 **Hand lotions and creams** A selection of fast-absorbing, extra-rich skin conditioners and lotions are also used for quick massages. Have a slow absorption rate if you intend to use as a massage medium.

2 **Foot balm** A richer, more emollient formulation is needed for the feet. Treatment ingredients like urea are essential if the skin is very dry.

3 **Sanitizer** A soap-free cleanser is used for removing residue and preparing the nail, as well as for sterilizing. There is no need to rinse.

4 **Skin exfoliating cream** Gently sloughs off dead skin cells from the surface of the skin, leaving it smother and cleaner. A slightly coarser formulation is preferred for the feet.

5 **Activator** Used to speed up the setting times of the resin after its application; it also helps ensure a strong bond. If too much accelerator is used or if it is sprayed close to the natural nail plate, a heat reaction might occur.

6 **Nail polish remover** Used to dissolve and remove nail enamel; usually contains acetone. Use acetone-free polish remover for artificial nails, as the acetone will weaken or dissolve tips, wraps, glues, and sculptured nail components.

7 **Cuticle creams and oils** Used to lubricate and soften dry cuticles and brittle nails; usually contains waxes and fat, such as lanolin, petroleum, beeswax, and cocoa butter.

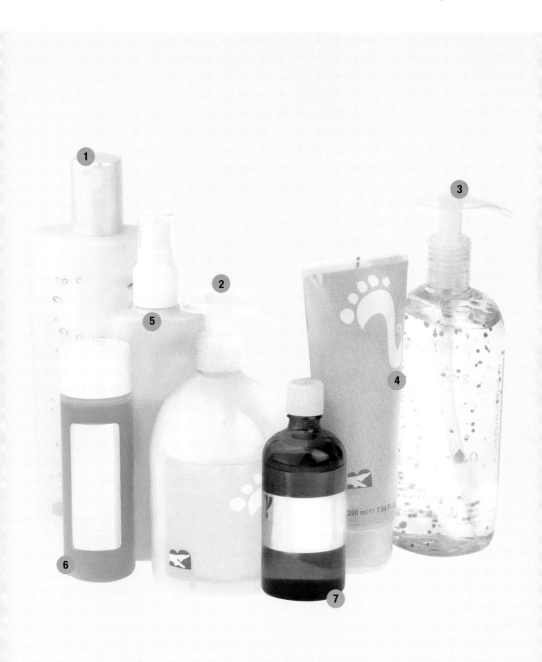

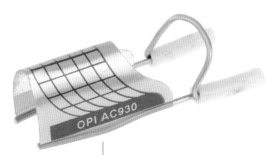

**Nail sculpting forms** These are adjustable supports, which are applied to fingertips under the free edge of the nail plate. The acrylic or gel is then applied to the nail plate and extended over the support to create an extension of the natural nail plate. Various forms are available, with and without printed guidelines, including sticky-backed foil, reusable metal forms, and plastic forms.

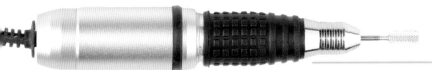

**Electric file** A big investment but makes short work of overlays and can be used to remove calluses and dry skin on feet, file down nails, and do buffing.

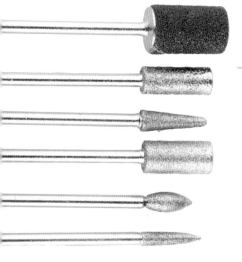

**Electric file bits** A variety of bits allowing various applications including filing, buffing, exfoliating, and shortening nails.

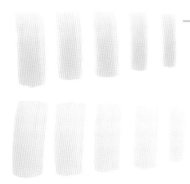

**Nail tips** Used with nail glue to extend a short nail. Usually the tip starts halfway up the natural nail and once glued in place will need to be reinforced with a gel, acrylic, or wrap overlay, or completely covered to extend the natural nail. Look for acrylonitrile-butadine-styrene (ABS) plastic as it's more flexible, more opaque, and easier to blend in, as well as adhering better. Acetate tips are more difficult to blend and won't bond as well with adhesives, nor will they create a convincing natural nail.

**Orangewood stick** Wrapped in cotton pad to push back cuticles and to clean underneath the free edge (instead of a nailbrush).

**Sable brushes** For applying acrylic monomers, polymers, and gels.

**Dappen dishes** Used to contain monomer liquids; their small size helps reduce the evaporation of product.

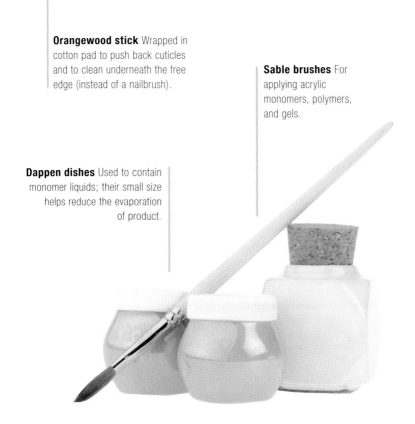

# Types of polish

**Ridge filler** A self-leveling formula that smoothes and fills the nail surfaces, creating a uniform, even finish.

**Basic base coat** Prevents dark shades of nail varnish from yellowing or staining the nail plate.

**Specialist base coat** Formulations are available for brittle nails as well as normal nails.

**Nail whitener** Available in pencil, paste, or cream form, it contains titanium dioxide or zinc oxide.

**Nail strengthener or hardener** Prevents splitting and peeling of the nail plate.

**Cuticle remover** Dissolves excess cuticle tissue on the nail plate. The active agent is usually 2–5% sodium hydroxide or potassium hydroxide with glycerine added as a humectant. The product is brushed on and left for a few minutes and then washed or wiped off. Because it has a high alkaline content, contact dermatitis can occur if the product is left on for too long. Cuticle removers can also damage and soften the nail plate; paronychial inflammation is common.

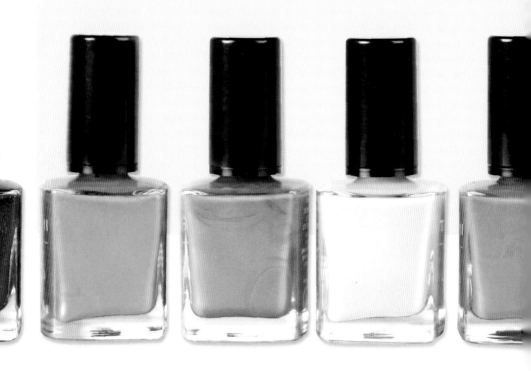

**Nail polish** Contains a solution of nitro-cellulose in a volatile solvent, like amyl acetate, and evaporates quickly. Manufacturers add castor oil to prevent it from drying out too rapidly.

**Top coat or sealer** Prevents chipping and adds shine to the finished nail. Usually contains nitrocellulose, toluene, a solvent, polyester resin, and isopropyl alcohol.

**Liquid nail dry and high shine** Speeds up drying time while adding a high-gloss finish with UV inhibitors and reflective polymers to prevent chipping, smudging, and yellowing.

**Liquid nail dry** 60-second drying; helps protect a fresh manicure and pedicure from scratching, smudging, and wrinkling, thanks to special film formers that protect the polish.

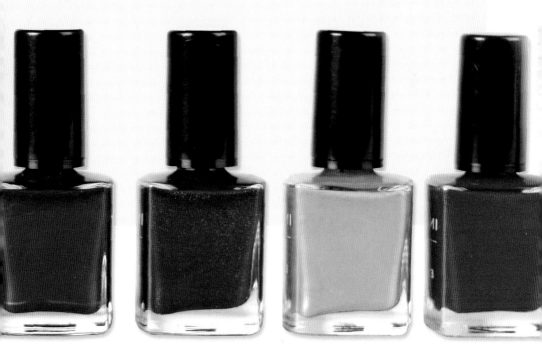

# Acrylic nail supplies

See Chapter 5 for further details on acrylic nail art.

**Gel products or light-setting gels** These contain a monomer, an oligomer resin, and a photo-initiator. The photo-initiator reacts with the light, triggering a molecular response, which hardens and sets the gel. Similar gel systems use either a spray-setting system, which uses a chemical initiator triggered by a spray chemical, or a brush-on activator system.

**Wrap systems** These include adhesives like cryanoacrylate glues, various fabrics like silk, fiberglass, paper or linen, and catalysts or adhesive setting sprays, which help reinforce breakages, acrylic tips, or weak nails.

**Fiberglass systems** These include a catalyst or setting spray to stabilize the product; fiberglass resin that contains a monomer and polymer and needs the catalyst to harden properly; and fiberglass fabric to reinforce and strengthen.

1 **Sculptured nail liquids** Like ethyl methacrylate, arc monomers—small individual molecular units, which can join together to form a polymer. Combining the powdered polymer with the liquid monomer creates a chemical reaction that hardens the product.

2 **Antistatic brush** For removing dust filings and debris from the surface of the nails.

3 **Pre-primer** Formulated to cleanse and dehydrate the nail plate and work as a preparing agent. Dehydrates and cleans, removing dust, contaminants, and oils from nails before applying finish gel or polish. You can also use acetone to the same effect.

4 **Tip cutters** Short-bladed, spring-handled clippers for cutting nail tips.

5 **Nail tips** Can be long, short, curved, straight, curved sideways, or flatter from side to side. The choice of shapes, plus around ten size choices, means that most natural nails can be fitted with a tip, but a variety of shapes and sizes are essential.

6 **Adhesive disposable forms** Probably the most widely used adjustable supports for sculpting nail extensions. Easily adjusted to fit all nail shapes.

7 **UV sealer** A special UV blocking top coat that protects pink and white nails from discoloration due to sun exposure or tanning.

8 **Protein bond** Adheres to the keratin structure of the natural nail and provides an anchor for gel, acrylic, and polish.

9 **Acrylic nail powders** Clear, natural, white, and pink.

10 **Dappen dishes** Small dishes needed to contain small amounts of polymer powders and liquid monomers when applying acrylic nails.

11 **Brush on glue** For applying tips—this formulation gives more control and dries within seconds.

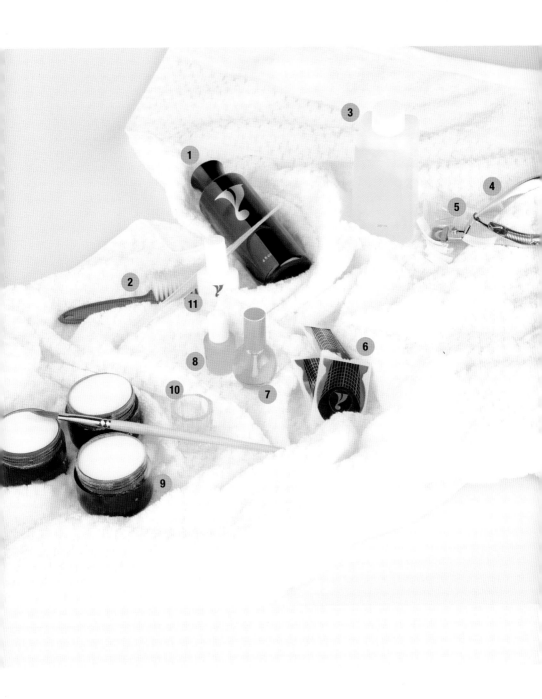

# CHEMISTRY

The nail industry cannot operate without the use of certain chemicals. Nail technicians will know how nail products work together on the nail; if you're going to attempt any of the more complicated procedures in this book at home, specific product knowledge provided by the manufacturers and suppliers will enhance your skills and understanding.

Once you get the hang of it, it's fairly simple really.

Here is a list of some of the more commonly used chemicals and terminology.

- **Acetone** A colorless, volatile, extremely flammable solvent that can be used safely for the removal of artificial nails and for dehydration of the nail plate. It can be very drying and irritating, depending on the frequency of use.
- **Acrylates** The family of monomers used in light curing gel products.
- **Acrylic** All of the main systems used contain monomers that are closely related; in fact, all systems are different forms of acrylic: cryanoacrylate—adhesives, wraps, and no-light gels; acrylates—UV light gels; methacrylates—UV light gels, monomers, and polymers.
- **Activator or accelerator** Used to accelerate or speed up the setting process of the resin; too much accelerator or activator sprayed close to the natural nail plate can result in a heat reaction.
- **Adhesive** A chemical that allows two surfaces to

bond together. Many of the adhesives used are cryanoacrylate.
- **Catalyst** A catalyst is a chemical that speeds up or slows down a chemical reaction. It is usually a weak alkaline solution that is brushed or sprayed on, causing an instant reaction.
- **Curing** The hardening or setting time a liquid will take to become solid.
- **Cryanoacrylate** An adhesive or "super glue" often used for tip application.
- **Cyanoacrylates** A branch of acrylics. The monomers from the branch are primarily used in wraps, no-light gels, and tip adhesives.
- **Ethyl methacrylate (EMA)** The most commonly used monomer in acrylic systems and the preferred ingredient for liquid/powder systems.
- **Formaldehyde** An ingredient used in some nail

polishes and glues; it is a known allergen and suspected carcinogen. Overuse will dehydrate the nail plate, causing splitting and flaking.

- **Formalin** A stabilized form of formaldehyde, often found in nail hardening products.
- **Free radicals** Quick-moving molecules that cause a chemical reaction.
- **Glutaraldehyde** A disinfectant that is not safe or appropriate for home use. Skin contact or inhalation of the vapors will affect your breathing and can cause serious allergic reactions.
- **Inhibitors** Ingredients that prevent monomers and/or oligomers from prematurely hardening or gelling while still in their original container.
- **Initiator** An ingredient within a product formulation that causes a reaction, the speed of which is controlled by a catalyst. In the gel system, the initiator is in the gel, which is activated by UV light. In fiberglass, the initiator is in the activator, which reacts when painted or sprayed on. In the liquid and powder system, the initiator is present in the powder—usually benzyl peroxide—and will react once the monomer is combined with it.
- **Methacrylates** A family of monomers used in liquid/powder systems.
- **Methyl methacrylate (MMA)** A monomer that is prohibited in many countries because it damages the natural nail when used in high concentrations as an artificial nail enhancement.
- **Molecule** A chemical in its simplest form; molecules that cannot be broken down any further are elements.
- **Monomer** Often referred to as the liquid part of the liquid and powder system. "Mono," meaning one, refers to a single unit or molecule.
- **Oligomer** A short, single chain of molecules— either a polymer with many molecules, or a monomer with a single molecule. Found in UV gel systems.
- **Polymer** Long chains of molecules linked together; while polymers can be liquid in the nail industry, they are usually solid in powder form.
- **Polymerization** Setting that occurs when a

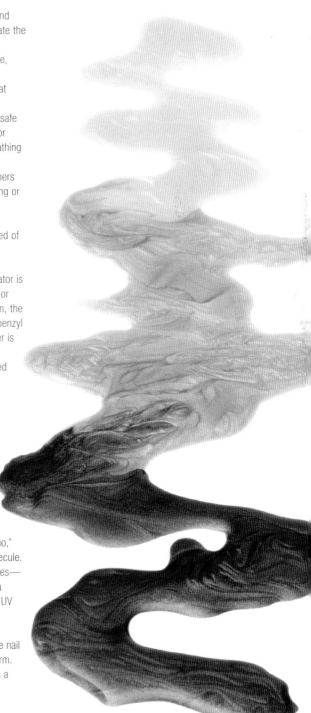

polymer and monomer are combined; an initiator, usually benzyl peroxide, is needed to start the reaction, as is a catalyst to control the reaction.

- **Primer** Usually methacrylic acid-based, primers are corrosive—so use sparingly and carefully. Useful for removing oil and bacteria and for dehydrating the nail plate.
- **Solute** A substance that is being dissolved.
- **Solvent** A substance that dissolves another substance.
- **System** Used in this context, refers to the three acrylics methods: liquid and powder, UV gel, and fiberglass.
- **Toluene** Obtained from petroleum and mainly used as a solvent. Similar to benzene but less volatile. It also maintains polish in liquid form until it is ready to apply.
- **Volatile** Describes a substance that evaporates or diffuses easily, for example at room temperature.

## Chemical reactions

We need to understand how some molecules bond naturally, while others, because of their positive or negative attraction, will need assistance in the form of heat, light, or an initiator to speed up the setting process. All systems need an initiator to start a reaction as well as a catalyst to control the speed at which the liquid turns solid. All acrylic processes require polymerization to turn a liquid or semi-liquid into a solid.

Chemical molecules can be arranged and rearranged into almost limitless combinations, and this rearranging of molecules is a chemical reaction. Some molecules can join together to form a long chain, called a polymer, or remain molecules by themselves (monomers). The liquid in the "liquid and powder system" is the monomer, and the combination with the powder containing the initiator creates a heat reaction that splits the initiator in half, resulting in two free radicals; each free radical energizes a monomer. Each energized

### Safety glasses

Wearing safety glasses is recommended, especially when clipping tips or working with chemicals. A splash of polish remover can be extremely painful, not to mention the damage potential of cuticle remover, wrap resins, tip adhesives, and acid-based primers.

monomer then attaches itself to another monomer, creating a chain reaction that results in the polymer chain being created. Too little powder can result in a soft and weak solid, while too much powder can result in a very hard solid that is too brittle. The correct ratio is crucial to the viability of the product; getting this right takes time, practice, and an experienced eye.

Gel systems are normally associated with oligomers. Similar to the monomer and polymer system, gels are supplied already mixed. They are placed on the nail and then cured under the UV (ultraviolet) light, which, in this case, is the initiator. While oligomers are chains of molecules, they are much shorter than polymers and allow the UV light to penetrate the gel, enabling curing to take place. UV gel is more sensitive to oxygen than the liquid and powder system, as oxygen inhibits the polymerization of the gel nail. UV gel always has a sticky layer after curing, which needs to be buffed off or polished. Viscosity varies greatly from product to product; thicker gels are more difficult to master and are prone to shrinkage, while thinner gels are self-leveling and better at retaining their shine.

# Proper disposal

It is important to consider where your unused chemicals end up. Products that were not designed to be flushed down the toilet or poured down the sink should always be properly disposed of. Flammable and corrosive materials should be stored in an appropriate and safe location until they can be disposed of. Check with the product manufacturer or distributor for the Material Safety Data sheet for information on proper disposal procedures.

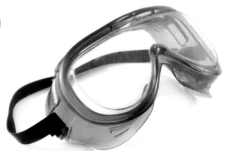

# Overexposure

For all chemicals there is a limit to the level of exposure that is deemed safe. When that level is exceeded, the body reacts; so early warning signs should never be ignored. Once an allergic reaction is experienced and you know the cause of the reaction, it is necessary to remove the irritant or product immediately. Many people wear thin rubber gloves to work in if they have had an allergic reaction to a product. Watch out for localized skin reactions, any redness or inflammation, and cuticles that become itchy or sensitive to pressure.

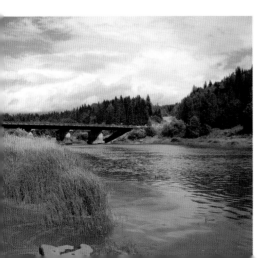

# Inhalation, absorption, and ingestion

There are three ways potentially harmful chemicals can enter the body. If these are prevented, then hazards can be avoided:

**1 Inhalation** Caused by breathing in the vapor or dust of the chemicals. Although not easy to control, with effective ventilation and care, it can be minimized. Overexposure through inhalation is a serious risk. While the nose has thousands of tiny hairs and mucous membranes to prevent foreign bodies being absorbed into the lungs, there is always the risk of respiratory problems.
Adequate ventilation is essential to avoid eye, lip, and nasal irritation. If you are a technician, this might necessitate investing in a specially designed extraction unit (by opening a door or window you are often just circulating vapor). Finally, be aware that just because you can't smell the vapors doesn't mean that there aren't any. To minimize inhalation, you need to ensure the following:

- When using a liquid and powder system, be sure you pick up the correct mix ratio each time; excess monomer wiped onto a paper towel will evaporate into the atmosphere.

- Spraying chemicals into the air increases the risk of skin, eye, and inhalation exposure, so control mists by avoiding pressurized cans. Look for nonpressurized pump sprays that create larger, heavier droplets that don't travel very far.
- Keep all products, bottles, and jars tightly sealed when not in use to prevent evaporation of product.
- Decant monomer into small containers for use; this will help minimize evaporation by limiting the exposed surface area.
- Use self-closing metal waste bins—plastic bins allow vapors to escape, thereby contaminating the air. Place all wipes and cotton balls into the bin after usage.
- Wipe up spills immediately with paper towels and dispose of them in an outside trash can.
- When using a solvent to remove artificial nails, cover the bowl with a towel to minimize evaporation.
- Also be aware when using an electric file that very fine airborne particles are easily absorbed, so a dust mask is a good idea. Dust generated by hand filing is denser and will fall onto the work surface, making it easy to dispose of.
- Discard all unwanted nail solvents and monomers by soaking them up in absorbent paper towels and placing them in an outside trash can; larger quantities should be placed in safe containers in the open and allowed to evaporate. Never pour down sinks and toilets.

Overexposure through inhalation is easily controlled by keeping vapor and dust away from your breathing zone—a 2-foot (60-centimeter) sphere around our heads from which all the air we inhale is drawn. Ventilation issues must be looked at carefully and, if you are going pro, effective systems should be sought. There are all sorts of ventilation systems available, from exhaust and extraction methods, to charcoal filters and fans. The best bet would be to contact a professional fitter of ventilation systems, who will measure and advise on the best possible course of action.

**2  Absorption** Probably the most common cause of problems is the absorption of chemicals through the skin or nail plate. You can help prevent chemical absorption by the correct and safe application of chemicals:

- Cover all cuts and abrasions prior to beginning any nail treatment.
- Leave a margin around the cuticle line when applying any nail overlays.
- Never apply a monomer without the polymer powder, as the nail plate will absorb the excess, causing problems later on.
- Avoid touching the skin with any nail product during application, regardless of the system being used.
- Avoid applying "wet mix" of polymer and monomer.

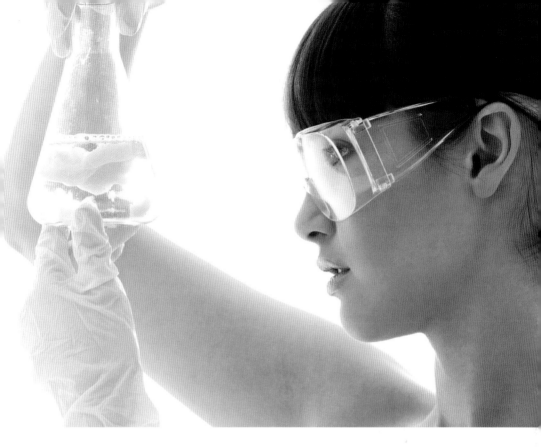

## Contact lenses

Don't wear contact lenses when working with nail products; the vapors can be absorbed into soft lenses, making them unwearable. This can seriously affect and even damage the eyes.

- Use the right brush when applying powder and liquid; a large brush can hold too much liquid, thereby affecting the mix ratio.
- Apply gels and fiberglass in thin, controlled layers, to aid curing.
- Change towels after filing as there is a risk of leaning in the dust, causing a skin reaction over time.

Allergic reactions are not always evident where you'd expect them to be—puffy and itchy eyes can sometimes be a reaction to product on the nails, while headaches, tiredness, mood swings, nosebleeds, and a sore throat can all be signs of a reaction to a chemical via any route of entry.

**3 Ingestion** Caused by chemicals entering through the mouth, ingestion is easy to control—it boils down to washing hands regularly and frequently, not eating or drinking around products, and following reasonable hygiene. Never drink hot liquids while working with chemicals; it's possible they could absorb vapors from the air or collect dust. Wash your hands before eating anything, as small amounts of dust and vapors are easily ingested.

# Hygiene

It is imperative to maintain fastidious hygiene methods, especially as there is always a risk of infection. All surfaces have the potential to carry microscopic pathogens, including your hands, the work surface, and the tools you use—even door handles and towels. Pathogenic bacterial and viral contamination is transmitted through direct and indirect contact; some germs are airborne and others can spread in water. Disease can be spread by direct contact with bodily fluids, like sneezing, or coughing, and with blood, pus, sores, cuts, and grazes. If you are working on someone else's nails, the only viral contaminants you need to worry about are spread by blood-to-blood contact as with hepatitis B (HBV) and the human immunodeficiency virus (HIV). Controlling all these risks is about awareness and decontamination before any eventuality occurs. There are three stages of decontamination:

## Sterilization

Eliminates all microorganisms—be they bacterial, viral, or fungal. Metal tools and implements like nippers and cuticle knives will need to be sterilized after use. If there is any contact with a break in the skin (even the smallest nick or cut) or with a nail condition, this process must be strictly adhered to. Sterilization is particularly important if tools have come into contact with bodily fluids like blood or lymph, as they could carry viral infections like hepatitis or HIV. Scrub all tools with soapy water or a solvent to remove any grease or debris, and then dry off carefully with disposable towels before sterilizing. Alcohol, gluteraldehyde, chlorine (bleach), and iodine are the main chemical sterilizing agents available. All are very strong irritants, so direct contact with the skin must be avoided.

## Disinfection

Will destroy some bacteria, viruses, and fungal spores, and will inhibit the growth of others. Use on hard surfaces and tools and equipment that don't come into contact with bodily fluids. Surfaces should be wiped down after every session; floors, light switches, sinks, and basins should be cleaned on a regular basis for general hygiene. Disinfection can be achieved by immersing implements in boiling water or steam, alcohol, methylated, or surgical spirits.

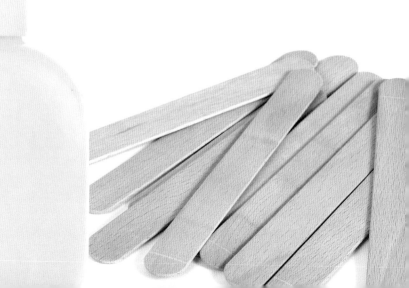

## Sanitation

Sanitation is probably the lowest level of decontamination and, in the case of nail preparation, it is essential to maintain healthy nails by removing traces of artificial nail products and dust. Get into the habit of washing hands before and after every treatment. Proper washing reduces pathogens and contaminants by 99 percent. Sanitizing significantly reduces the amount of pathogens and other contaminants considered safe by health professionals. Be aware that pathogens can grow on soap and in soap dishes, so it's best to use a liquid soap. Pay particular attention to the underside of your nails, where a scrubbing brush is most useful. Be sure to remove all traces of soap with lukewarm water, and use an alcohol-based sanitizer.

# Hygiene tips

- Wash and sanitize hands before and after each manicure.
- Wash down all surfaces regularly.
- Sterilize all metal tools and disinfect all implements after each manicure.
- All cuts and abrasions must be covered with a bandage to avoid secondary infections.
- Files and buffers used in any treatment should either be disposable or personal; disposable items offer the preferable solution.
- Avoid using sharp instruments on inflamed or infected skin.
- If you have direct contact with another person's blood or body fluid, wash the area with soap and hot water as soon as possible.
- Choose pumps or sprays for creams and lotions, or use a disposable spatula—when you dip your fingers into a container of lotion or cream you add bacteria to it.
- If you have any obvious infections, do not reuse cuticle creams, moisturizer, or polish.

# Chapter 3

# MANICURE AND PEDICURE BASICS

What could be more relaxing and comforting than having a manicure or pedicure? There are different types of manicures and pedicures—try combining the basic with a different treatment each time, including mask, paraffin wax, hand and foot massages, reflexology, spa treatments, and acrylic nails.

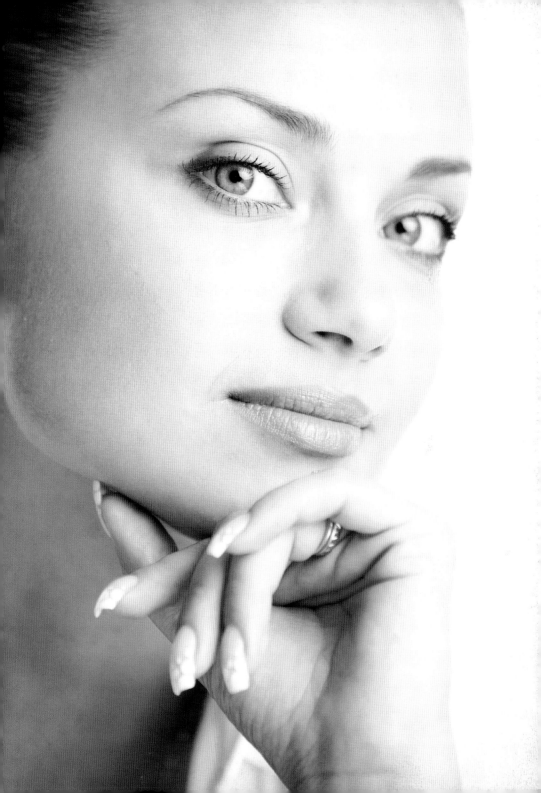

# SHAPING THE NAIL

When selecting your preferred nail shape, you will need to consider the shape of your natural nail, your lifestyle and occupation, and finally the structure and shape of your natural nail plate. If you're keen on sports, have young children or work with your hands, shorter nails will be a more practical solution than long nails.

It's the sides of the nail that give the nail plate its support. If the sides are filed away to give the nail a narrower look, the support is lost and the nail is considerably weakened. The maximum length shouldn't be longer than the length of the natural nail plate. It is best to file your nails only when the white part of the nail—the tip—has grown 0.2 inches (half a centimeter) from the nail's stress point, where the free edge meets the pink part of the nail plate. Filing your nails before this point will weaken them. If you are looking for a natural-looking shape, look no further than the nail bed. Observe its natural shape, and shape the tips accordingly. Basic shapes include oval, almond, round, and rectangular or square.

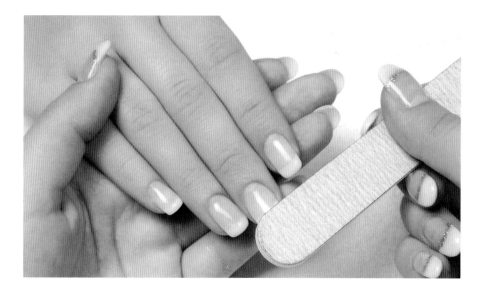

## Oval

Filing the nail plate into an egg shape is ideal for thick or wide nails; feminine and flattering, it is ideal for short and mid-length nails.

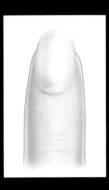

## Almond

Filed away at the sides and softly pointed at the tip to resemble an almond, this nail shape can make the fingers look fat, so avoid it if you want to grow out the length of the nail.

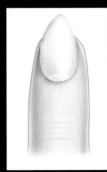

## Round

Ideal for the shorter nail; softly rounded at the tip, strong, and neat; best suited for short nails and most men.

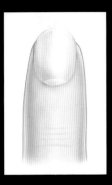

## Rectangular or square

Allow the sides to grow straight forward without shaping, then file the tip straight across at right angles to the rest of the nail. Popular for very long nails and for people who work with their hands. Short, square nails tend to make hands look blunt and heavy.

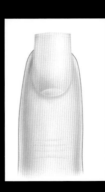

## Square with rounded corners

Softer and prettier than severely squared nails.

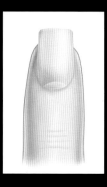

## Oval with squared off tip

Useful for narrowing a too-wide nail; the squared-off tip adds strength.

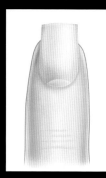

## Straight-sided

With the nail slightly rounded at the tip, this shape is allowed to grow straight forward and the tip is gently rounded at the end. This is the strongest shape with maximum support from the sides.

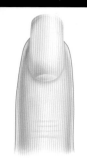

## Pointed

Filed into a point; this nail will break easily and is unflattering and old-fashioned.

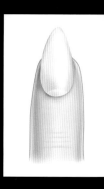

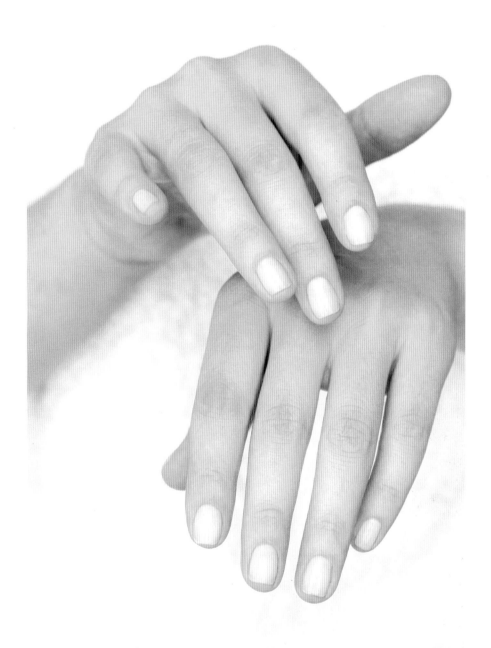

# MANICURE AND PEDICURE

There are many products available for you to choose from; each manufacturer will have their own manicure products and methods for you to try. Whether you are giving yourself a manicure, or treating a friend to one, create a relaxing environment before you start and have all your supplies ready and organized. You can try using a luxurious paraffin wax or hot stone massage before you start, or add a gorgeously scented aromatherapy massage, or an indulgent mask to your basic routine—all these extra touches will add to your overall manicure experience.

## Manicure essentials

**Basics** A comfortable chair, good lighting, towels, a metal wastebasket with plastic liner and a lid, sterilizing solution and sterile container, a manicure bowl—a glass fingerbowl specially shaped for soaking your fingers in warm water—and antibacterial soap.

**Supply tray** To contain your products, such as polish removers, cuticle creams, surgical spirits, nail dry oil, top coat, base coat, ridge filler, nail strengthener, creams and lotions, and finally a good selection of colored nail polishes.

**Implements** Cuticle nippers, nail clippers, nail scissors, cuticle pusher or knife, natural nail buffer, nail brush, files and buffers, emery boards, and plastic spatula or tongs (for removing product from its container, as using your fingers increases risk of contamination).

**Disposables** Disposable paper towels, cotton balls, lint-free pads, orange sticks, and tissues.

See pages 46–9 for your basic manicure equipment.

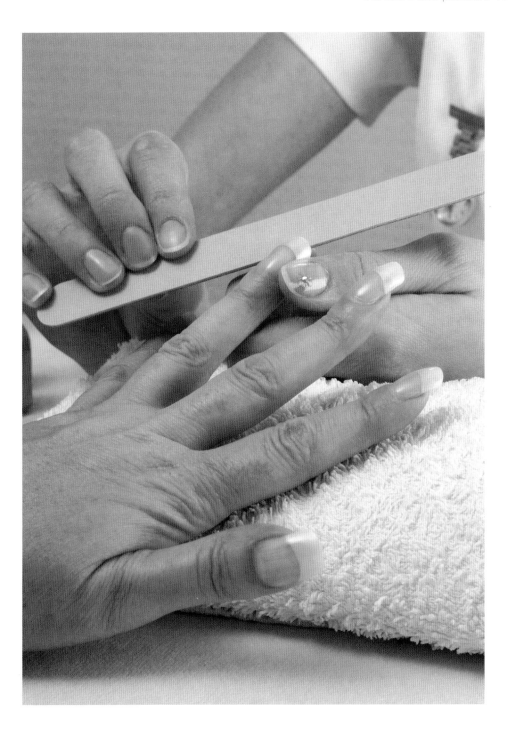

# Time needed for different types of manicures

The time it takes to do a manicure depends not only on the type of manicure, but also on the condition of your nails and the expertise of the person performing the manicure. The following are rough guidelines only.

| | |
|---|---|
| Basic manicure and single color polish | **30 minutes** |
| Traditional French manicure | **45 minutes–1 hour** |
| American manicure | **45 minutes–1 hour** |
| Paraffin (or luxury) manicure | **at least 1 hour** |
| Hot stone manicure | **at least 1 hour** |
| Spa manicure (with aromatic salt rub) | **1 hour, 30 minutes** |
| Regular manicure, acrylic nails | **1 hour, 15 minutes** |
| Regular manicure, UV gel nails | **1 hour, 15 minutes** |
| Regular manicure, elaborate nail art | **up to 2 hours** |

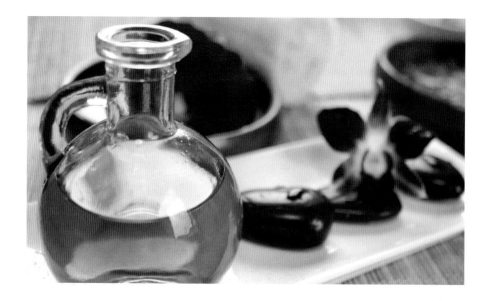

# Pedicure essentials

**Nail file** For shaping and filing toenails.

**Sanitizer** or antiseptic foot spray. Usually contains antifungal and antibacterial agents.

**Nail clippers** Two types are available. To avoid curved nail plates shattering, clip the nail in two parts, first one side and then the other, after soaking the nail in warm water to soften.

**Files** For removing dry skin and calluses.

**Foot mask** A luxurious addition and, depending on the formula chosen, has many therapeutic benefits such as boosting circulation and eliminating toxins. Apply with a brush and simply peel off when done.

**Cuticle oil** To soften and nourish dry cuticles and make the nail plate more flexible.

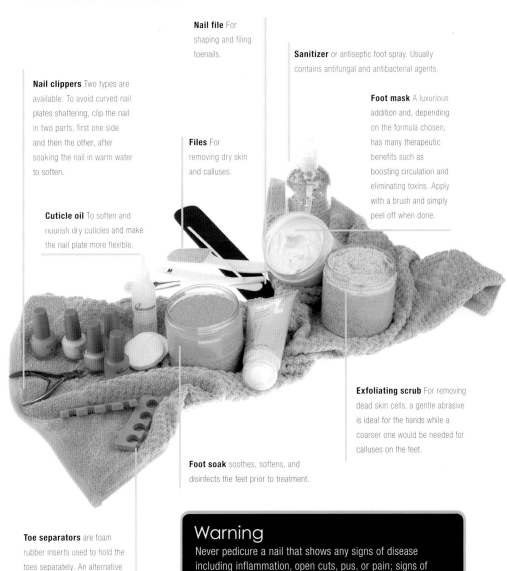

**Exfoliating scrub** For removing dead skin cells, a gentle abrasive is ideal for the hands while a coarser one would be needed for calluses on the feet.

**Foot soak** soothes, softens, and disinfects the feet prior to treatment.

**Toe separators** are foam rubber inserts used to hold the toes separately. An alternative is cotton wool pads, which can be wound between the toes to separate them.

# Warning

Never pedicure a nail that shows any signs of disease including inflammation, open cuts, pus, or pain; signs of bacterial or fungal infection, which presents itself as a brownish green or white discoloration and crumbling of the nail; or shows signs of common flat warts (which are caused by extremely contagious viruses).

# Basic manicure step-by-step

There are numerous products on the market and some suppliers might suggest a different sequence. But this is a basic manicure and you can personalize it by including a paraffin wax or hot oil procedure to make it more specialized. With all the new spa treatments around, you can really get creative.

## step 1

Before you start, ensure that you are comfortable, warm, and relaxed. Have all your products ready and your working area prepared. Remove jewelry and check for any possible fungal infections, open cuts, or any areas that might need special attention such as hangnails.

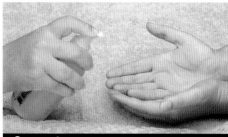

## ⊕ step 2

Sanitize the hands; depending on the product you're using, you could simply spritz, soak the hands, or wipe them back and front with a cotton pad soaked in sanitizer.

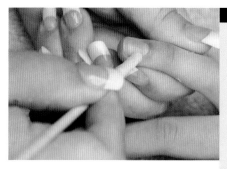

## ⊖ step 3

Remove polish—soak a cotton pad in remover, then hold it over the varnish for a few seconds before stroking it off the nail toward the free edge. If you are wearing artificial nails, use an acetone-free remover to avoid damaging them. If you are right-handed, start with the left hand, working first on the thumb, then the index finger, middle finger, ring finger, and finally the little finger. Then move to the right hand, starting with the thumb, then the little finger, ring finger, middle finger, and finally the index finger. Reverse the process if you are left-handed. An orange stick covered with cotton can be used to remove all remaining traces from around the cuticles and the sidewalls, and under the free edge.

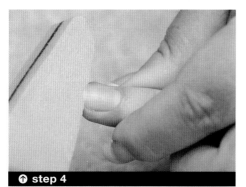

**⬆ step 4**

Shape the free edge of the nails. After you have chosen the desired length and shape, file the natural nail with an emery board, keeping the file at a 45° angle to create a beveled edge. The roughest side of the emery board is drawn across the nail. File from the right side to the center of the free edge and from the left side to the center of the free edge; avoid filing into the corners of the nail. Then run the smooth side across the nail downward over the free edge, again at 45°. Avoid using a sawing motion, as this will cause tearing of the nail. File each hand, working from the little finger to the thumb.

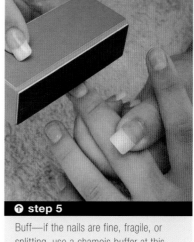

**⬆ step 5**

Buff—if the nails are fine, fragile, or splitting, use a chamois buffer at this stage. Buff the nails in one direction only—from the base of the nail to the free edge, making sure to lift the buffer after each swipe to avoid heat buildup. Small imperfections or unevenness can be gently buffed away. See page 96 for more information on buffing.

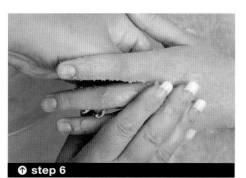

**⬆ step 6**

Exfoliate—apply a mild exfoliator or scrub to dampened hands, and gently massage. Exfoliation sloughs off dead skin cells, buffs away dullness, boosts circulation, and leaves the skin primed and ready for the next product. Rinse off hands and dry thoroughly.

## Pro Tip

The larger the number, the smaller the grit particles; the larger the grit size, the smoother the surface finish you will achieve. White plastic buffers can be washed and disinfected, while a chamois buffer is better for home use.

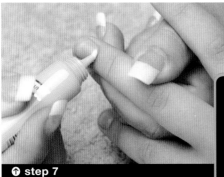

**↑ step 7**

Soften the cuticles—apply cuticle cream either directly from the cuticle cream tube or with a cuticle stick, then massage into the nail plate, nail wall, cuticle, and down the first joint of the finger, using the pad of your thumb in a firm circular motion.

## Pro Tip

Cuticles: always push back cuticles gently. When you feel the skin resisting, it's time to stop; if using cuticle knives, work with water or oil for lubrication to prevent the tools scratching the nail plate. Don't leave the cuticle remover on for too long, as it has a very dehydrating effect on the skin. Be very careful to remove only excess cuticle and not to remove any living skin, as this could cause bacterial infections and contamination.

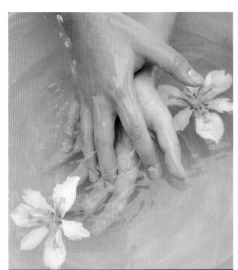

**↑ step 8**

Clean the nails—place hands into a bowl of warm soapy water and soak for a few minutes. Remove and dry thoroughly with a tissue or towel.

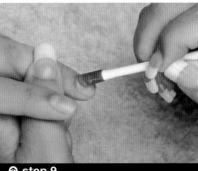

**↑ step 9**

Apply cuticle remover—using an orange stick covered with cotton to clean under the free edge, push back the cuticles, and remove any nonliving tissue from the nail plate with a gentle circular motion. Hangnails will need to be trimmed at this stage. Wipe or wash off any remnants of cuticle remover or loose skin.

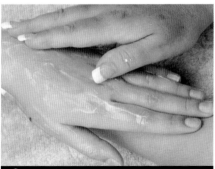

**↑ step 10**

Apply massage cream, lotion, or oil to hands
and gently massage into the skin.
(See massage routine on pages 88–93).

**➔ step 11**

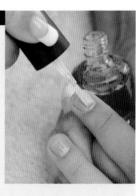

If nail polish is
being applied,
you will need to
remove all
traces of oil,
cream, or lotion
with a non-oily
nail varnish
remover. Follow
by wiping with
water to
remove any
solvent; this will ensure proper polish adhesion.
Use nail polish remover and lint-free cotton pads
to wipe each nail prior to varnish application.

**➔ step 12**

**Polish application** Polish the nails using one
base coat, two coats of preferred nail color, and a
top coat. If you are using a pearlized polish, you
might need three coats, depending on the desired
effect. Complete coverage on the first coat of
color will depend on the consistency of the nail
polish being used. Use very thin coats and build
up coverage rather than trying to correct polish
application with multiple strokes. As the solvent
evaporates, the coating becomes sticky and
impossible to work, so aim for as few strokes as
possible for a really professional finish.

**Base coat** It is essential to use a base coat,
because it contains an adhesive resin, which helps
adhesion to the nail plate by forming a barrier,
preventing staining by the colored pigments found
in some darker polish formulations. The base coat
is a milky, matte formulation that settles into the
ridges, leveling the nail plate. Make sure the base
coat is completely dry before applying colored
polish, or peeling and bubbling may occur.

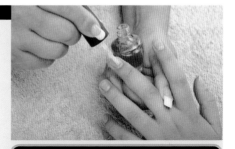

## Pro Tip

To get the right amount of polish on the
brush, the first time you remove the brush
from the bottle do it slowly, using a swirling
movement. As you swirl, press all sides of
the brush against the neck of the bottle,
removing excess liquid as you pull the brush
out of the bottle. If you don't do this, a blob
of polish will gather on the shaft, flooding the
nail plate and ruining your manicure.

# Basic polish application

**Prepare nail plate** All traces of creams, lotions, or oils must be removed from the nail plate before polish application or the polish won't adhere and could peel. First, wipe the nail surface with a non-oily nail polish remover, then wipe with water to remove any last traces of solvent.

**Prepare polish** Ensuring the correct polish consistency is crucial; the solvent ingredient in the nail polish is volatile, which means that the solvents keeping the polish fluid evaporate quickly when exposed to air. If a bottle remains open during application, or if it is exposed to extreme heat,

## Pro Tip

The bottle of nail polish should be rolled between the palms of your hands; vigorous shaking may causes air bubbles and will not give a smooth finish.

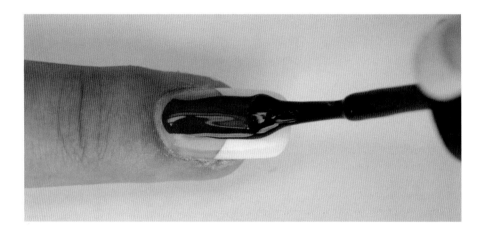

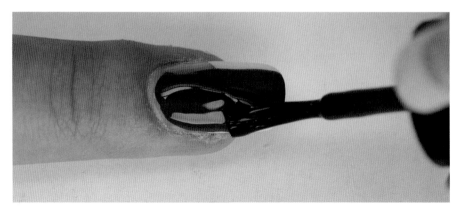

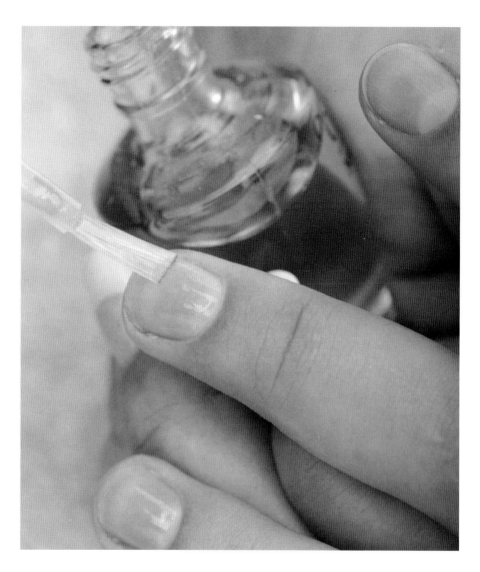

the solvents will quickly evaporate, ultimately resulting in thick, gooey, and stringy enamel. Be sure to keep your nail enamel bottles tightly closed when not in use. Store polish in a cool, dark place and keep the neck of the bottle clean to prevent any clogging and thickening. Nail polishes can be thinned with a solvent or a mixture of solvents that form the same base as the enamel, but make sure you use a thinner developed by the same manufacturer as the nail polish to avoid any problems. Never thin down your nail enamel with nail polish remover; it contains oil, water, and other impurities, which could prevent the polish from hardening properly.

**Polish application** The same application technique is used for the base coat, colored nail enamel, and the top coat, although slight variations

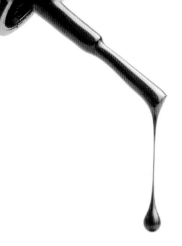

might occur, depending on the width of the nail plate and the shape around the cuticle.

To get the right amount of polish on the brush the first time you remove it from the polish, take the brush out of the bottle slowly, swirling the shaft of the brush up against the neck of the bottle to remove all the polish on the shaft. When the end of the shaft is reached, press the brush up against the far side of the neck of the bottle; there will be enough polish on the brush to cover the nail plate. When necessary to replenish, just dip the brush, but not the whole shaft, and repeat the last movement to withdraw it.

Place the brush three-quarters of the way down the nail plate, then gently push the brush forward up to the cuticle, allowing the brush to create a straight line and then brush toward the free edge in a long straight line. Hold the brush at a slight angle downward so that the polish is spread using the longer length of the brush, to help control and ensure even, smooth application—just make sure you reach all the way from the cuticle to the free edge in one stroke. Subsequent strokes are applied to either side of the first stroke—keep strokes to a minimum; the more strokes you make, the more lines or unevenness will result. Most polishes will need two coats to cover evenly, and frosty or pearlized formulations might require a third coat.

**Touch-ups** Keep the rounded end of a cuticle stick standing in a container of nail polish remover to attend to any touch-ups you might need to do. If you get nail polish on the cuticle, use the cuticle stick to remove it, then take the stick from the remover, tap it onto a tissue to remove any excess liquid, and use it to wipe away any polish on the skin. Use one wiping motion to avoid spreading the stain. Don't leave this clean-up process until the polish has dried; it is more resistant when dry so work nail by nail for efficiency.

**Quick-dry** A variety of products is available to help speed up the drying time of nail polish.
These include sprays and dry oils, which help ensure any scuffs slide off the surface of the nail without making an impression. They also help to condition the cuticles. Don't use the quick-dry between layers, as it will make the polish bubble and peel. Hot-air dryers are not a good idea either, as the forced drying can result in your manicure chipping or the polish fracturing.

**Peeling and bubbling** Usually the result of incorrectly prepared nail surfaces, or a base coat that has not been allowed to dry sufficiently. It can also occur if nail drying products have been used between coats of polish, or if layers of polish are too thick.

**Maintenance** This is essential if you want to protect and retain your primed hands. Here are some home maintenance tips:
● Regular application of cuticle oil will help keep cuticles in good condition and prevent them overgrowing onto the surface of the nail.
● Always wear rubber gloves when washing dishes—soaking your nails in water is the surest way to weaken them. Detergents strip the natural

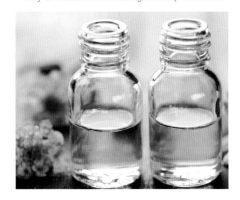

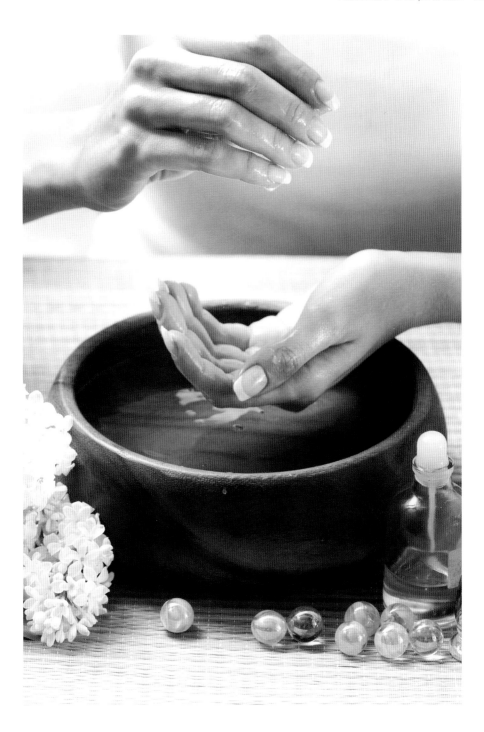

## Nail polish application methods

1 Full coverage—the entire nail plate is polished.
2 Free edge—the free edge is left unpolished to prevent nail polish from chipping.
3 Hairline tip—the nail plate is polished and a millimeter of polish is removed from the free edge to prevent nail polish from chipping.
4 Slim-line or free walls—leave a millimeter margin on each side of the nail plate to create a narrow, slimmer effect.
5 Half-moon—the lunula at the base of the nail is left unpolished and gives the illusion of shortening the nail.

- If your hands are very dry, try massaging them with plenty of treatment cream or warm oil last thing at night. Wear a pair of cotton gloves to prevent bed linens from being soiled and to ensure thorough absorption of the lotion.
- Maintain your manicure by applying a clear top coat to nails every other day to prolong your nail polish, brighten it up, and prevent it wearing away at the tips. This will also ensure added strength and protect the nail plate.
- The fastest way to prevent soft, weak nails is to apply a hardener once or twice a week; it not only saves vulnerable nails but also gives nails a high-gloss sheen.
- Never scrape off nail polish, as this can scrape off the protective cells of the nail surface. Peeling off flaking nail polish can also be very damaging.
- Unless your nails are very long, avoid clipping them to shorten them as this can cause them to bend or split. Rather, use an emery board to file nails down to size. Filing straight up against your nail can peel the tip, so hold the emery board at a 45° angle under the free edge.

oils from your nails. Also wear gloves for gardening chores to prevent damaging your hands.
- To prevent age spots, get into the habit of wearing sun protection, especially when driving.
- Get into the habit of applying hand cream every time you wash your hands to help boost moisture levels and minimize brittle and dry nails. Keep a pump dispenser of hand lotion by every sink in the house.

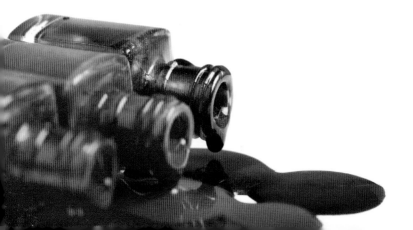

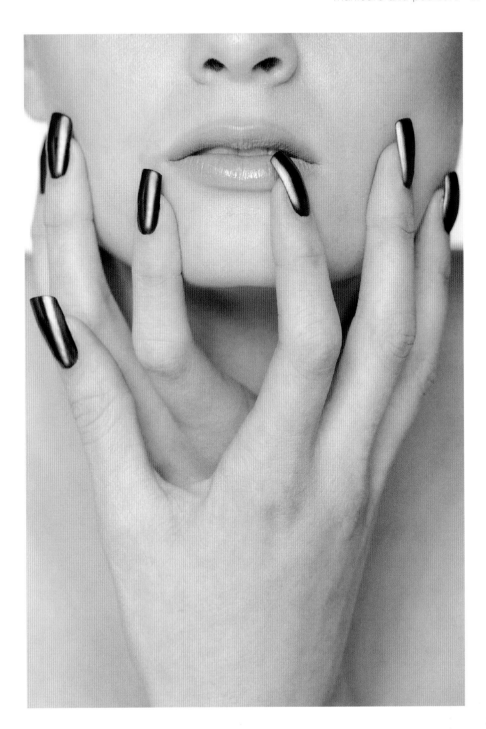

# MASSAGE

One of the oldest forms of healing, massage is the ultimate de-stressor—great for relaxing tired muscles, stimulating lymph drainage, and improving circulation. Massage also helps relieve pain in tense and rheumatic muscle fibers. Nodules and muscle spasms are smoothed away, resulting in a tremendous sense of well-being.

You can draw upon a variety of massage disciplines including reflexology, Swedish massage, acupressure, and Shiatsu, to develop your own techniques. Without a doubt, a masterful massage can transform an ordinary manicure into an extraordinary experience.

There are numerous massage routines and, with time and practice, you will discover your own favorite. Find the ones you are most comfortable with and practice until you have a massage routine that flows without your having to think about it. If you are massaging someone else, make sure you adjust pressure and style according to their preference. And be confident; there is nothing worse than being on the receiving end of an insecure and unconfident massage.

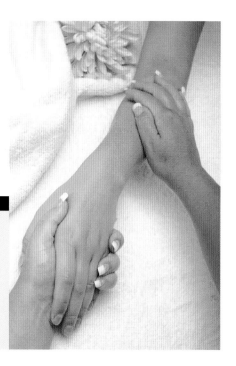

### ❷ step 1

Warm the massage medium in your hands, then apply using long stroking movements from the elbow to the fingertips. Begin by using the effleurage movement (see page 92), stroking your hand up the front of one arm and gently come down the back of the arm. Apply pressure going up and releasing the pressure as you come down. Repeat a few times on both arms and hands.

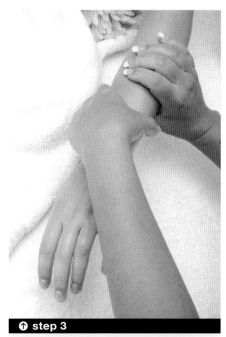

### ⬆ step 2

Moving your thumb(s) in a circular kneading motion, move up the front of the arm to the elbow, slide arms back down, and repeat a few times. Make sure that you are not being too vigorous or applying too much pressure.

### ⬆ step 3

Use petrissage movements next. This is a stimulating or kneading movement (page 92) that increases the blood flow as you lift the muscle at the side of the arm, gently lifting away from the bone. Use the palm of your hand and, in large circular movements, work toward the elbow. This stimulates circulation and relaxation and helps release the toxins. Repeat this 3 times on both sides of the arm.

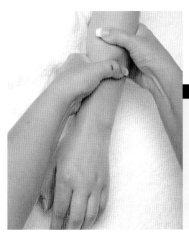

### ⬅ step 4

Then place thumb(s) on the arm so they are horizontal, and move them in opposite directions, from wrist to elbow and back down to the wrist. The squeezing motion moves the flesh over the bone and stimulates the arm tissue. Repeat 3 to 5 times.

### ● step 5

With your palm down, support the wrist while applying gentle pressure to the muscles of the upper arm, using the inside of the knuckles. Holding the hand, palm facing down, position your thumb(s) on top of the hand with the rest of your fingers underneath the pads of the palm. Massage in this position then turn the hand over so that your thumbs then work the pads of the palm. Use friction movements around the elbow area and slide your hands down to the wrist. Repeat this movement.

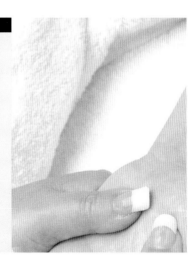

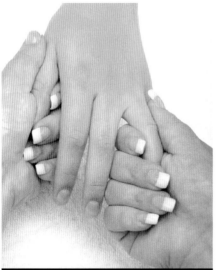

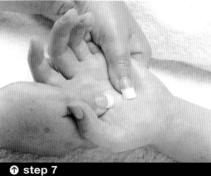

### ⬆ step 7

Lift your arm to the upright position with the palm turned upward. Apply thumb effleurage to the metacarpal spaces, linking this with small thumb circles starting at the wrist and working toward the elbow. When you reach the elbow, slide back down to the wrist and begin again; repeat 3 to 5 times.

### ⬆ step 6

Holding the hand palm down, push the hand upward and, using the thumb(s), gently press in a clockwise direction, moving over the entire palm as you work. Repeat for the other hand.

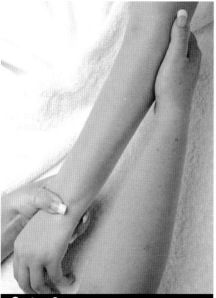

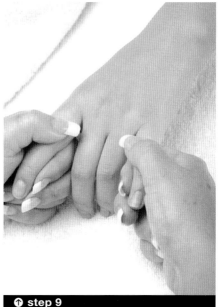

### ↑ step 8

Cup the elbow with your right hand and rotate your hand over it using a friction massage movement. Do this 3 to 5 times. To finish the elbow massage, move your left hand to the top of the forearm from the elbow to the fingertips as if climbing down a rope. Repeat 3 to 5 times.

### ↑ step 9

Turn the hand back over and slide to the little finger. Holding it at the base of the nail, gently rotate, working outward, repeating 3 to 5 times on each finger. Circle the joints one by one and then gently rotate the finger. Pull gently down the length of the finger to the end of the tip.

### → step 10

Effleurage up the entire hand and arm to the elbow a few times. Each time apply slightly less pressure. To end the massage, take each hand in turn and stroke either side.

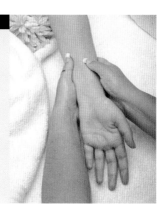

**Effleurage** Usually the first massage movement in any massage routine, it can consist of very light stroking movements or much heavier ones, depending on the amount of pressure applied. Effleurage massage is given by applying pressure in one direction using the palm pads on the flat of the hand—always toward the heart to aid venous and lymphatic flow. The hands and fingers are always returned to the starting point with light contact.

**Petrissage** is a technique that includes kneading, rubbing, or rolling the muscle to stimulate circulation, relaxation, and the release of toxins. More vigorous than effleurage, it must be slow and rhythmic. The muscle is gently lifted away from the bone, stretched, squeezed, and released. The most common toxin in muscles is lactic acid, a by-product of our cellular respiration processes, especially during times of muscle overuse when our natural detoxification systems cannot keep up. The benefits of petrissage include increased circulation, improved lymph movement, and better muscle tone.

**Vibrations** are fine tremulous movements of the tissue, done with the fingertips or the whole hand. The movement is along the course of a nerve and can restore and maintain nerve and muscle function. The manicurist's hands and arms must be fully relaxed and then contracted to produce the vibration movement, which is either static or running.

**Friction** is created by making small circular motions with the balls of the thumbs, fingertips, knuckles, and even elbows. These movements push the muscles against the bone, breaking up nodules or adhesions in the underlying tissue, rather than the surface of the skin. Stand over the area to be treated and use your body weight to penetrate the deeper tissues. The deep movements relax, aid circulation, tighten, tone, and assist in breaking up fibrous tissue.

# Pro massage and reflexology tips

Avoid massaging anyone in the following circumstances:

- Contagious or infectious skin disease—an increase in the venous and lymphatic drainage will encourage spread to other parts of the body. There is also the risk of spreading infection by contact.
- Internal inflammation, such as arthritic inflammation or swollen fingers and joints—massage can worsen the condition over inflamed areas.
- Varicose veins—pressure on or below these might cause further dilation, thrombosis, and the formation of varicose ulcers.
- Hairy areas—can cause irritation, rash, and discomfort.
- Recent wounds or scars—risk of stretching scar tissue; any pressure will disrupt normal healing processes.
- Any unexplained lump, swelling, or severe pain—these should always be investigated by a qualified medical practitioner.
- Any bruised areas—this will cause pain and will damage underlying tissue, possibly causing ulceration and delaying natural healing.
- Slow-release injections or patches—massaging around these areas could cause increased release of the drug leading to overdosage.
- Fractures—pressure over fractures would cause pain and interfere with natural healing processes; can result in exaggerated calcium deposit formation, causing future problems.
- Neuralgia or neuritis—if inflammation or pain is present, massage will aggravate and irritate the condition further.

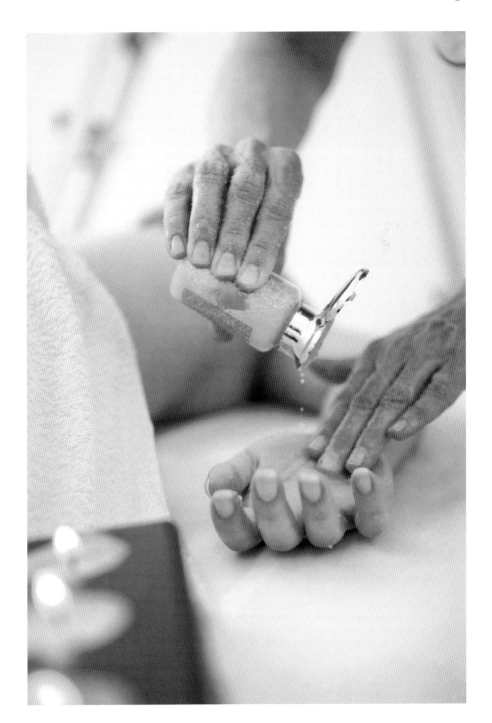

# ADDITIONAL TREATMENTS

Besides the basic manicure, there are various different treatments available to suit your age, lifestyle, and hands.

## Men's manicure

Basically the same as a woman's manicure, except that nail polish will not be used, although some men enjoy a clear matte polish. Buffing is an important part of a man's manicure. If nails are yellowed, you can bleach them with a prepared nail bleach or by applying 6 percent hydrogen peroxide.

## Electric manicure

The electric manicure is done with a small portable machine with a motor, which looks a bit like a drill. It uses a variety of attachments, including an emery wheel, cuticle pusher, brush, and nail-buffing disk. Be careful not to apply too much pressure at the base of the nail with the cuticle pusher and buffer.

## Hot oil manicure

Ideal for dry skin and cuticles and helps moisturize dry, flaky, or brittle nails. Warm some oil in a small bowl inside another bowl of hot water—or use a specially designed temperature-controlled oil heater to heat up the oil.

## Paraffin wax

Initially used by doctors as a therapeutic treatment, paraffin is a petroleum by-product that has excellent heat-sealing properties. Most waxes are a blend of paraffin and beeswax and are highly flammable. Solid blocks of paraffin wax are melted into a liquid, then maintained at a temperature of around 120°F. The treatment is ideal for boosting the circulation, improving skin condition, relieving the pain of arthritis and rheumatism, and for deep-cleansing the skin.

## Child's manicure

A child's manicure can start off with simple hand sanitation followed by nail filing and shaping. Soaking the nails softens the cuticles for treatment and then the nails are cleansed and buffed or polished. Little girls adore pretty pastel shades, sparkly, clear, and glitter nail polish. Daisy chain patterns applied to a transparent polish is a fun idea, but check with mom first!

# Paraffin wax

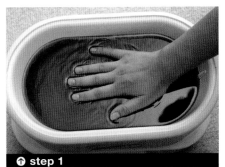

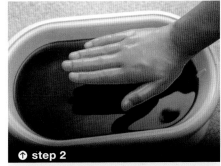

**⬆ step 1**

Apply a nourishing oil or cream to the hands or feet. Test the temperature first, then immerse the whole hand or foot into the wax bath, fingers spread apart.

**⬆ step 2**

Remove the limb from the wax, wait 5 to 10 seconds for the wax to solidify, then immerse again.

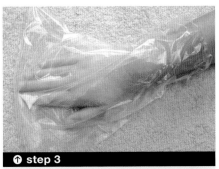

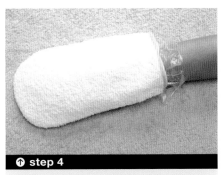

**⬆ step 3**

Repeat until the limb has been dipped 5 to 10 times, then place into a plastic bag, or wrap in plastic wrap.

**⬆ step 4**

Finally wrap in a warm towel for 10 to 15 minutes or until the wax loses its heat.

**➔ step 5**

Unwrap and peel off the wax and discard it after use. You can finish the treatment by massaging in the remainder of the nourishing oil or cream that you applied before dipping the hand into the hot paraffin. The hot paraffin ensures deep penetration of nourishing creams, oils, or lotions.

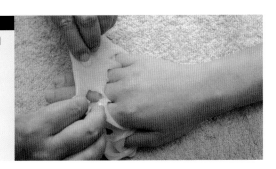

# Nail buffing

Buffing rids the nails of ridges and jagged edges and helps increase blood circulation to the nail bed.

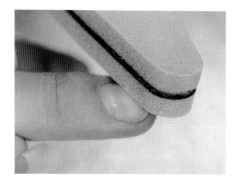

## Chamois buffers

The old-fashioned way of buffing is usually done with a slightly abrasive paste polish, mainly used on natural nails. The abrasive quality of the paste used with the buffer smooths the nail surface, giving it a shiny finish. It also helps bind the nail layers together at the free edge, which is very beneficial for flaking nails. With nail paste, it is important to buff from the matrix toward the nail tip so that the paste is not pushed into the cuticle. Be sure to lift the buffer from the nail after each stroke to prevent heat buildup on the nail surface. Just remember, the natural nail bed has few nerve endings to work as heat receptors, so once you feel a heat reaction it is too late—always try to work lightly and gently when buffing.

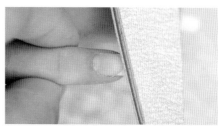

## ● Graduated buffer files

Buffer files are now available in a variety of materials and are used specifically to achieve a high-gloss shine and a smooth nail surface. Use the soft to medium grit emery board when smoothing or removing stains or nail glue sticking to the nail plate—a coarser grade emery can file away the natural nail before you know it. As artificial nails grow away from the cuticle with the nail plate, glues and buffer files are used to smooth and seal the join between the artificial nail and the natural nail plate.

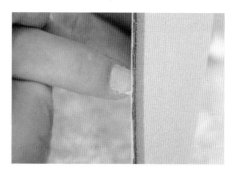

## ● Buffing natural nails

If you are buffing natural nails, you need to use a buffer rather than a low-grit file, as these are only for use with nail enhancement products. Position the buffer down the nail and not across, and buff in one direction using light movements, from the top of the nail to the bottom and then diagonally, creating an "X" to ensure the whole nail plate is shiny. Repeat around 10 to 12 times maximum; be sure to lift the buffer after each stroke to avoid excessive heat buildup.

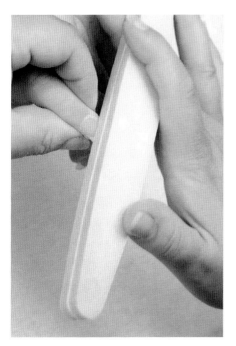

### ➊ Buffing nail enhancements

The files and abrasives you use will depend on the nail system you are using. A great technician will be able to create great nails with a minimum of filing. To ascertain how much filing you need to do, look at the nail from its top view, side view, and down the barrel or "C" curve. Work out where you need to file away any bulk, as this will need a lot of buffing. Make sure you use a rounded motion so you're working with the right curves. Once you have refined the shape so that the nail is thin at the cuticle and free edge and thickest at the apex, or where the flesh line is visible, you can then buff the entire nail using a high-grit file or buffer. Check the highlight under your lamp, ensuring a continuous straight line all the way down the nail.

## Buffing overlay to repair broken nails

Broken nails are usually the result of rough treatment or having used one's nails as a tool. Long nails need to be treated as if you have just applied a fresh coat of nail polish—being longer means they are weaker than "normal" nails, and therefore require TLC.

If the nail is torn off and only a small amount of length is lost, filing the other nails to match is probably the best option. If, however, the remaining nail is very short, a tip and overlay or a sculptured extension would be your best bet. Using a tip, overlay it with a wrap material like paper, silk, or fiberglass, a thin layer of liquid and powder, or a layer of gel to produce a repair that can grow right out with the nail. Keep the overlay very thin at the cuticle, and as the nail grows and you return for manicures, simply buff the overlay and shorten it accordingly. Try to keep the overlay as thin and natural-looking as possible. If the product is applied too thickly, an old repair will get "tip heavy" as it grows out, and then the natural nail won't be able to support the tip, which will result in cracking and breaking along the stress line. To avoid this happening, try to maintain repairs, and as soon as nail growth allows, file out the original crack and remove the false nail product from the nail surface. Keep the nails at an appropriate length by filing your fingernails regularly.

# THE FRENCH MANICURE

Probably the most requested treatment of all nail enhancements, this neutral nail looks clean and healthy and suits all occasions. It also creates the ideal foundation for most nail art applications. You can combine it with other artistic designs like flowers, pearls, rhinestones, and lace.

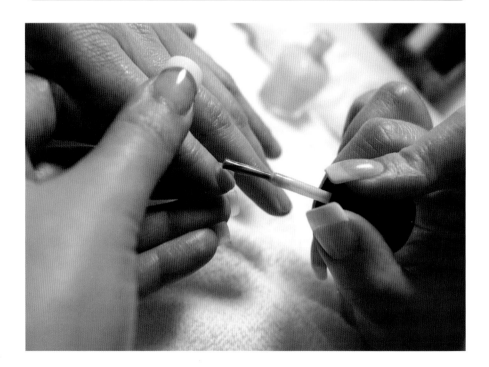

A French manicure can make a short nail look longer and slimmer if done correctly. The easiest method is probably the airbrush method, using a stencil, but this is expensive to set up. Freehand application is quick and simple to do with a little practice. To get it right, the nails will need a free edge. Very short nails are impossible to do. Your nail polish should not be thick and sticky and you need a very steady, practiced hand.

- Apply your base coat.
- Apply white polish to the free edge of the nail, starting on the left and sweeping the brush across and down to the bottom right-hand corner—this creates a sharp chevron effect. Repeat on the other side.
- If a rounded, smile effect is wanted, swipe the brush across the nail, dipping it slightly to achieve a curve.
- Apply clear, sheer pink, peach, or natural polish over the entire nail using the 3-stroke method as before.
- Apply a top coat over the entire nail.

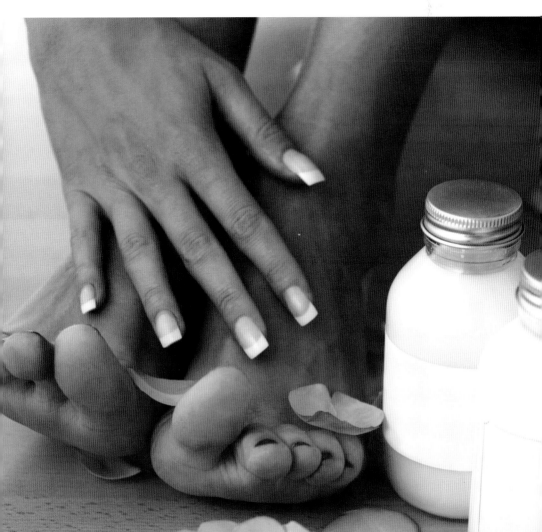

# French manicure

The French manicure is one of the most popular nail treatments used to enhance the natural beauty of the nails—a standard procedure at many nail salons worldwide. This look is achieved with a neutral or transparent pink-colored polish on the whole nail, with white polish on the tips. The French manicure is a great base for nail art; of which there are endless variations such as pearls, rhinestones, and striping tapes. With acrylic nails, there are tinted acrylic powders that can be applied for the same result.

**➔ step 1**

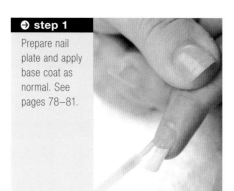

Prepare nail plate and apply base coat as normal. See pages 78–81.

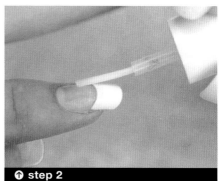

**⬆ step 2**

Using the nail tip color, usually white, create a tip to the free edge of the nail by starting at one side, usually the left side, and sweep across toward the center of the free edge on a diagonal line. Repeat this on the other side. This will create a "V" shape, which can be left just like that or, if you prefer, fill the open top of the "V" by sweeping across the center of the tip to create an even sweep of the white polish and a more convincing finish.

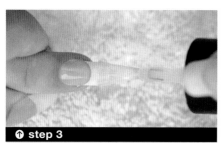
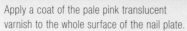

**⬆ step 3**

Apply a coat of the pale pink translucent varnish to the whole surface of the nail plate.

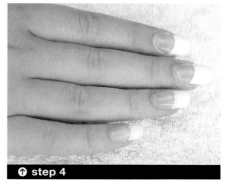

**⬆ step 4**

Apply top coat over the entire nail plate.

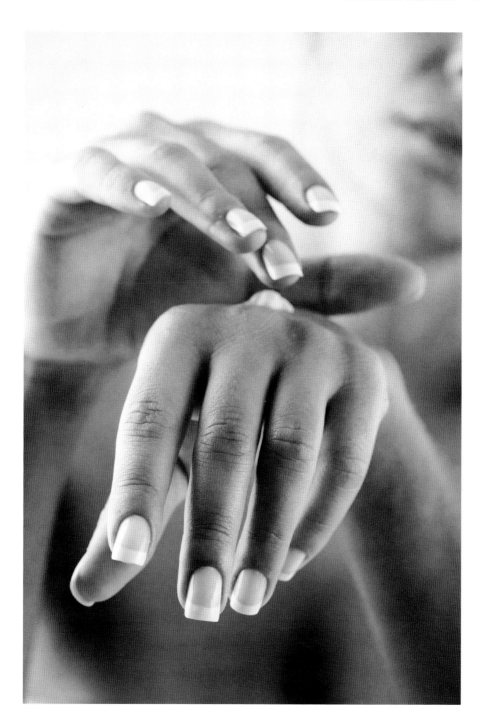

# French, American, and English manicures

There are many types of manicure style, just as there are many different fashion trends. Practicalities often play a large role in the popularity of some of these trends. For instance, what could be more practical than a "no polish" polish? This explains the popularity of the French manicure; easy to wear every day, it is neither ostentatious nor obvious, plus it won't clash with what you're wearing. It also lasts far longer, makes the nail look clean, healthy, and very pretty, and doesn't show up wear and tear like a darker shade would do.

The most popular style of manicure in France, for example, is different than the most popular style in America or England. Painted nails are, after all, a fashion statement, and fashion trends have always differed around the world. The French, in particular, are renowned for their sense of style, their sartorial *savoir-faire*! It's not surprising then that the traditional French manicure is still the most recognizable and popular nail fashion statement. It helps that it's one of the most affordable too.

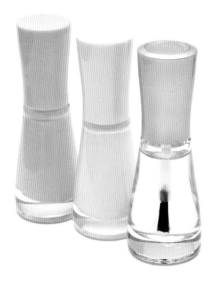

## The French manicure

The classic elegance of French fashion is reflected by the simplicity of the French manicure. The French manicure consists of a white tip—the free edge—and a flesh-toned sheer top coat over the rest of the nail. The look was first made famous by Jeff Pink of French beauty brand Orly in 1975 (though its origins can be traced back to the 1930s when Max Factor created the look for Paris "fashionistas").

Soon afterward, the look was introduced onto the fashion runways of Paris, where it became an instant classic. From that point on, this iconic look became known as the "French manicure." Love it or hate it, if you're planning to become a nail technician you will need to master it. But remember—nails will need a free edge, varnish must not be thick or sticky, and you will need a steady hand unless you have mastered the air-brush (In which case a stencil makes all the difference).

The nail tips are painted the whitest of whites and a clear top coat is used. For the traditional French manicure, the strong white tips are always painted first and a natural, sheer top coat applied after. Moreover, the look is very versatile and suits all kinds of outfits, whether casual or formal. Some women, however, find this look very overpowering and prefer one that is a bit more toned down; they prefer the look of an American manicure.

## The American manicure

Also known as a Beverly Hills manicure, the American manicure is a softer look than the French, ensuring creamier colors as opposed to the stark white contrasted tip of the French manicure. The white tips are polished in a softer, more muted white and the nail beds are a pinkish, neutral color, with an almost nude, pale pink base color. In an American manicure, the tips are painted first and then the neutral shade, or light pink shade, is applied on top of it. The result is a look that is simple yet glamorous.

Becase of this, most people consider the American manicure to be a more natural nail. However, it also has many more variations than the French manicure. An American manicure (known in some countries as an English manicure) is not

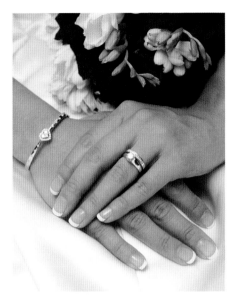

particularly Dita Von Teese. This is one look worth emulating on either long or short nails. Bear in mind, however, that the look does create the optical effect of shortening the nails.

- Prepare the nail plate with one coat of base coat.
- Paint the entire nail plate with a coat of white varnish and allow to dry.
- If you don't have steady hands and are doing this on yourself, look in your stationery drawer for some adhesive paper reinforcements—the ones you use to strengthen punched holes. Place on the nails so they block out a small arch, or simply line up with your natural lunula. You could try doing this freehand, but this method is so simple it is worth using.
- Apply two coats of deep red polish and allow it to dry thoroughly before removing the adhesive stickers.
- Apply a top coat to the entire nail plate.

restricted to a rigid color scheme of white tip and neutral overcoat. Basically, the major difference between the two styles is the color of the tip. Sometimes red is used on the tips instead of white or cream, and the rest of the nail is often painted in a stronger pink shade, as opposed to nude. The final difference between the French and American manicures is to do with the shape of the nail. The French look tends to favor a more rounded edge, which mirrors the natural curve of the person's finger. The American manicure is squarer, creating a bolder look which is seen as a more noticeable fashion statement. Both the French and the American manicures are extremely popular with brides, despite their subtle differences. This is probably because both looks adhere to the idea of sophistication and elegance that women strive for, especially on their wedding day.

## Half moon

This method of nail polish application was made popular in the 1940s and 1950s because it saved on nail polish. This method of varnishing involves painting the nail plate but leaving the lanula (half-moon) free of polish. It is very fashionable and is currently adored by all 1940s-inspired fashionistas,

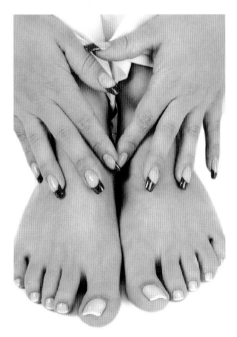

# PEDICURE

Feet are often neglected, hidden away under layers of socks in winter, or squashed into tight stockings and uncomfortable shoes all year round. Often neglected, they definitely need a little special care. When you book a pedicure treatment, be sure to take along a pair of open-toed shoes, or if the weather doesn't permit, make sure enough time is allowed for thorough drying, or follow these simple steps in the comfort of your own home!

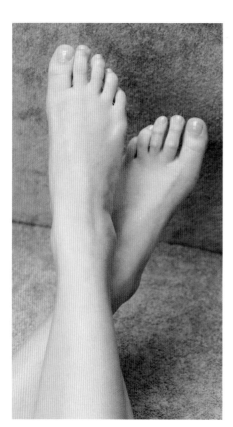

## Pedicure supplies

Foot soak, massage oil or lotion, cuticle cream or oil, polish remover, polishes (including base and top coat), toe separators, sanitizer, toenail clippers, emery board, pedi file (foot rasp), orange stick, corn and callus trimmer, toenail brush, foot powder, foot scrub or exfoliator, foot mask (optional), and foot cream. See pages 46–9 and 77.

# Basic pedicure step-by-step

### step 1

Disinfect or sanitize the feet and legs with an antiseptic solution and check for any contraindications.

### ➔ step 2

Remove all traces of nail enamel and place both feet into a soak for 5 minutes. This will help to soften the skin. After you finish soaking, remove one foot, and towel-dry.

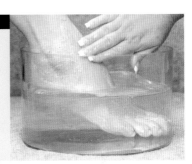

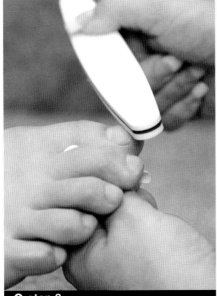

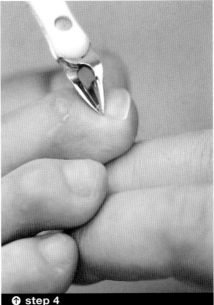

### ⬆ step 3

Clip nails to the required length. Don't try to cut across in one motion, as this might split the nail. Then, using an emery board, file across the top of the nail. Any corners should be filed away to prevent ingrown nails, then bevel at a 45° angle and smooth as you would a fingernail. Repeat on all nails.

### ⬆ step 4

Apply cuticle cream and gently coax back cuticles. Using a cuticle knife or pusher, remove any dead skin around the cuticles and lateral nail folds, trimming away any hangnails in the process with a pair of nippers.

### → step 5

Apply an exfoliator or foot scrub by gently massaging in circular motions over the ball and heel of the foot. Rinse off the scrub in the footbath, being sure to remove all traces of the exfoliant, then pat dry.

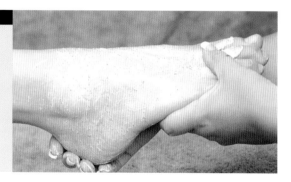

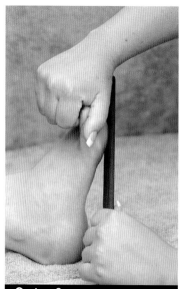

### ↑ step 6

Use a pedi file or foot rasp to remove any hard skin, being careful to avoid any soft areas of the sole. Repeat steps 4 to 6 on the other foot. To keep warm, keep the first foot wrapped in a towel while working on the other.

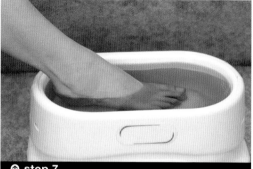

### ↑ step 7

You could introduce the paraffin wax treatment at this point. Prepare a paraffin wax bath as per the manufacturer's instructions, paying close attention to the correct temperature, immerse your feet one at a time, wait 5 seconds and repeat 5 to 8 times. Place feet in a plastic protector, and wrap in toweling mitts or hot towels. Leave for 10 minutes. Unwrap, peel off wax, and dispose of it.

### step 8

Massage the feet, ankles, and lower legs following the basic massage routine (pages 113–15).

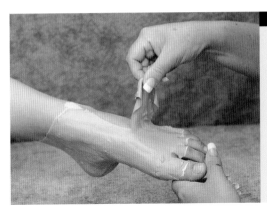

### ◉ step 9

A specialized pedicure mask (an optional alternative to the paraffin wax) is then applied using a brush; wrap feet first in plastic and then a towel to boost moisture and warmth. Hot towel compresses can be used to remove the mask unless you are using a peel-off variety, which is low maintenance and allows you to avoid yet another dunk into water.

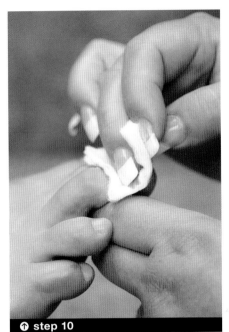

### ↑ step 10

Rub the nails thoroughly, ensuring all traces of lotions and exfoliants are removed in preparation for your polish application.

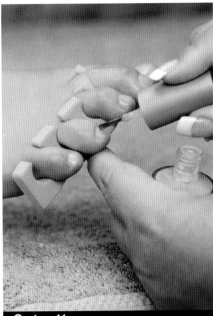

### ↑ step 11

Disposable toe separators are placed between the toes and a base coat is applied, followed by two layers of color and a final top coat. Allow 10 to 30 minutes drying time, depending on the varnish used, before removing the toe separators. If you must wear shoes soon after a pedicure, wearing an open-toed pair will help to prevent smudging.

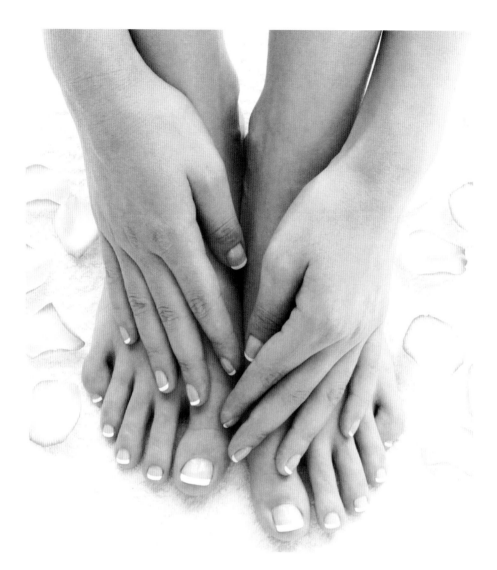

# Toenail shape and length

The toenail should always be square with the corners slightly rounded so that no sharp edges are left to dig into the nail wall. Never file the sides of the nail away; this will only lead to ingrown toenails or pressure pain at the sides of the nail as the nail plate grows forward. The most common problem podiatrists treat is ingrown toenails or onychocryptosis. Most ingrown toenails are self-inflicted, usually as a result of incorrect trimming techniques; trauma such as stubbing your toe; or from wearing tight-fitting shoes, socks, or tights that push the toe against the nail so that it pierces the skin. Try the tips on the following page to prevent this painful affliction:

- Cut toenails straight across so they are even with the tip of the toe. Rounding the corners may be prettier, but this only encourages nails to grow into the surrounding skin. Do not cut too short, too low at the edge, or down the side. File any pointed edges smooth with an emery board.
- Avoid using nail clippers because the curved cutting edge may cut the flesh. Nail scissors can also slip, so it is best to use nail nippers. These have a smaller, more manageable cutting blade and longer handles for ease of use.

- Cut nails after a bath or shower when they are softer and easier to cut.
- Rotate your footwear so that each pair of footwear has time to dry out thoroughly before you wear them again. Opt for breathable material and wear natural-fiber socks. In summer, wear open-toed sandals whenever possible.

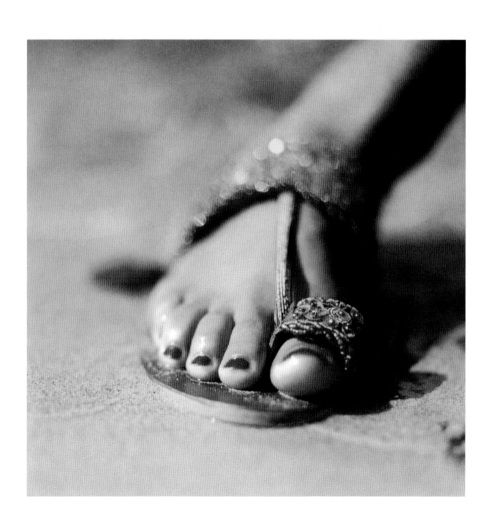

# Home care for feet

Toenails and feet need regular care to prevent problems and to maintain their appearance. Regular monthly pedicures will keep feet and toenails in good condition.

- To prevent odor and infection, feet should be washed and dried thoroughly every day. Lightly apply foot powder to keep feet dry.
- Regular use of a cuticle cream or oil will moisturize and maintain cuticles and surrounding skin, especially if feet are prone to dryness.
- Don't let your toenails get too long, especially if you wear shoes that are closed in at the toes. They could catch and press on the inside of the shoe, which can result in the nail lifting away from the bed. This is often seen in athletes, particularly runners.
- Keep hard skin in check by using creams or pumice stones.
- To prevent bunions or toe and nail deformation, shoes, socks, tights, and stockings should never be too tight.

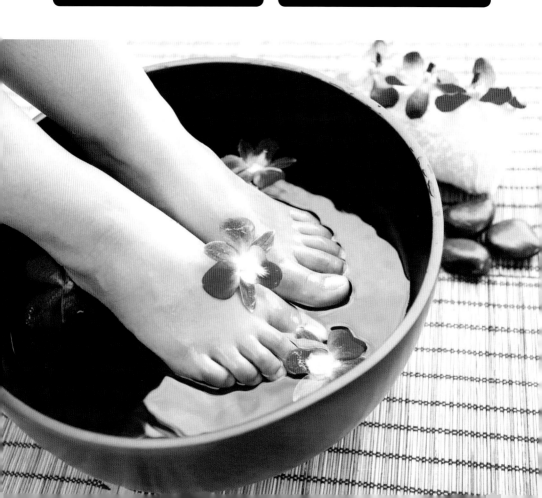

# Foot massage techniques

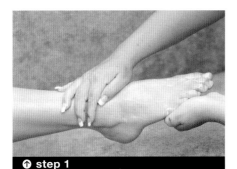

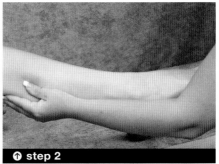

**↑ step 1**

Rub oiled or creamed hands together vigorously to warm them before beginning the massage. With the sole of the foot resting on your knee so that the leg is bent, use effleurage movements (page 92) from the back of the ankle. Apply slight pressure on the way up and stroke lightly on the way down. Repeat a few times. Using both thumbs, applying friction up the side of the shinbone to the knee; repeat a few times.

**↑ step 2**

Apply petrissage movements (page 92) with the palm of your hands up the side of the leg in circular movements. When you reach the knee, slide your hand down and repeat on the other side of the leg. Repeat on both sides a few times.

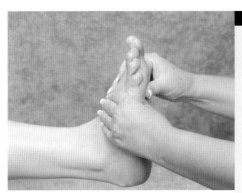

**← step 3**

Holding the foot, begin a long, slow stroking motion with your thumbs on the top of the foot, starting at the tips of the toes and sliding all the way to the ankle; then retrace your steps back to the toes with a lighter stroke. Repeat a few times. Now stroke the bottom of the foot with your thumbs, working in a scissor movement across the foot, starting at the base of the toes and moving from the ball of the foot, over the arch, to the heel and then back again.
Use long, firm strokes, and slightly press the sole with your thumb as you stroke. Repeat a couple of times.

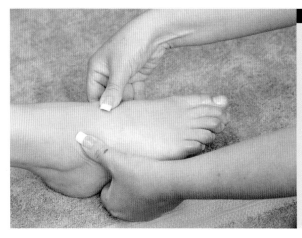

### ⊖ step 4

Friction movements (page 92) are now applied between the metatarsals on the upper surface of the foot, with pressure directed toward the heart. Follow this with a sliding pressure between the metatarsals.

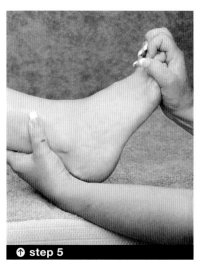

### ⬆ step 5

Friction movements are also applied to the joints of the toes, and the toes are then pulled to stretch the joints.

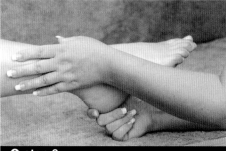

### ⬆ step 6

With your thumb and forefinger, move up the Achilles tendon with a gentle pressure. Cup one hand under the heel behind the ankle to brace foot and leg. Grasp the ball of the foot with the hand and turn the foot slowly at the ankle a few times in each direction. These rotations will help minimize stiffness, especially for those who suffer from arthritis.

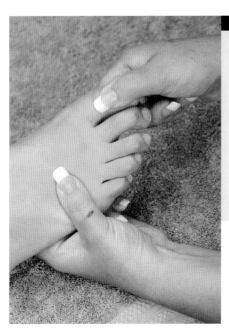

### ● step 7

Support the foot beneath the arch with the other hand, and beginning with the big toe, hold the toe with the thumb on top and index finger beneath. Starting at the base of the toe, slowly and firmly pull the toe, sliding your fingers to the top and back to the base. Repeat, but gently squeeze and roll the toe between your thumb and index finger, working your way to the tip and back to the base. Repeat these two movements on the remaining toes.

### ● step 8

Hold the foot behind the ankle, cupping it under the heel. With the index finger of the other hand, insert your finger between the toes, sliding back and forth a few times; repeat this movement between each toe. Then, using the heel of your other hand, push hard as you slide along the arch from the ball of the foot toward the heel and back again. Repeat a few times. Thumb and finger frictions should also be applied around the whole ankle joint, both front and back.

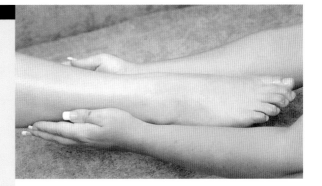

### step 9

Finish the massage by repeating a few vertical and sideways effleurage movements up to the knee, then bring your hands down, stroking the foot at the top and on the sole, and bringing your hands together to finish.

## Troubleshooting tips

1 If you have petite hands and fingers, your nails will look better filed to a more oval edge, which matches the natural shape of your fingers. If you have heavy-set hands and wide nail beds, a squared edge works best.

2 Buffing your nails to a high shine can look just as good as using a clear polish. It's also less time-consuming.

3 It's a good idea to invest in a good, double-sided nail buffer. Use the rough side to smooth away ridges and discoloration. Use the other side to smooth and shine the nails.

4 If you're using an oil massage medium, make sure that all traces of oily residue are removed thoroughly when dehydrating the natural nail and before any extension products are applied.

5 Whether you're receiving or giving a manicure, make sure any fiddling in bags for car keys is done before the final polish application. This will avoid smudges and smears in the fresh polish.

6 For perfectly filed nails, start at the edges and move toward the top. Only ever file in one direction!

7 Soak your hands in soapy water for a few minutes to soften the cuticles. Use an orangewood stick to push them back. Do not cut your cuticles, as this can cause infections and nail damage.

8 After moisturizing, remember to wipe your nails with a damp cloth to remove any excess oils. Your polish will then last longer and won't chip as easily.

9 Try to find a calcium gel base coat. Calcium will strengthen the nails and help them grow faster.

10 You should be able to cover your nail with your chosen nail polish in just three strokes, one on each side and then one in the middle. Apply two coats for a more vibrant finish!

11 Top coats improve wear by coating the polish with a protective shield. Fast-drying top coats tend to cause bubbling and uneven, dull surfaces. Best results are achieved with longer drying times.

12 Cotton swabs are not a good idea for cleaning up nail polish, as tiny microscopic threads can ruin your manicure. Instead, place a wooden orangestick into the nail polish remover and use it to clean up the area around the nail.

13 Never shake your nail polish. If you need to blend the polish, roll it gently between your hands.

14 To fix chipped polish, the best thing is to remove the polish and start again. If nail polish is prone to chipping, it could be due to the following: not using a base coat; nail polish was force-dried; polish was applied too thinly; incorrect nail preparation, or polish was thinned down or diluted.

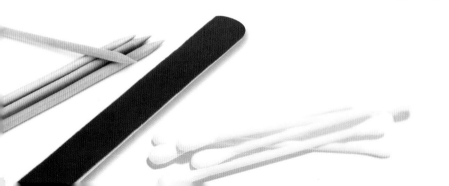

# Hand and finger exercises

At some point, most of us will experience some stiffness and aches resulting from overuse of the joints. To keep hands flexible, try taking a break from repetitive tasks and stretch your hands and arms several times to relieve tension. Here are a few exercises to help stretch your muscles, limber up your joints, and boost circulation, which in turn will improve the color and tone of the skin and increase the growth and strength of the nails.

1 **Fist fling** Clench both fists tightly, hold for 5 seconds, then spring open and stretch wide. Hold the stretch for 5 seconds before releasing. Repeat 6 times.

2 **Vertical lift** Holding your hands gracefully, palms down, lift up slowly from the wrist, then drop the wrist down. Keep the hands very relaxed but not totally limp. Move in circles first in one direction, then in the other. Repeat 6 times.

3 **Wrist shakes** Hold your arms out in front of you with the hands hanging limply. Then shake the hands up and down as hard as possible in a floppy movement, and then relax. Repeat this movement 6 times.

4 **Finger spread** Hold your hands up in front of you, palms down, fingers pressed tightly against each other. Now thrust your fingers apart, opening them as wide as possible. Repeat 6 times.

# Flexibility and movement

We often use our hands and wrists in vigorous and repetitive ways. Over the years, too much time spent repeating one task can take its toll. Look after your hands, vary the work that you do, and take care to avoid the problems listed below:

## Occupational Overuse Syndrome or Repetitive Strain Injury

This covers a range of conditions with symptoms that indicate discomfort or persistent pain in the muscles, tendons, and soft tissue. Caused by unsuitable working conditions involving forceful or repetitive movements, or by maintaining constrained or awkward postures such as those experienced by musicians or factory workers. Symptoms include swelling, numbness, restricted movement, and weakness in or around muscles and tendons of the back, neck, shoulders, elbows, wrist, hands, or fingers. Sometimes it becomes difficult to hold objects or tools in the hands, affecting one's ability to function at work and at home.

## Carpal Tunnel Syndrome

This is usually caused by pressure on the meridian nerve in the wrist, which causes pain, numbness, and tingling, or partial paralysis in the thumb, index, and middle fingers of the affected hand. It results from a narrowing of the carpal tunnels, the passages through which the nerves pass between the arms and hands. This condition usually affects people who use their hands a lot. The pain tends to worsen at night and increases over several weeks. Try to avoid movements that cause tenderness.

## Epicondylitis

This condition is accompanied by tenderness and pain in the muscles and tendons around the elbow. Often referred to as tennis elbow, but caused by repetitive motion.

## Tenosynovitis

An inflammation of the tendons and synovial capsules of the wrist and finger joints that makes movement of the hands and wrists very painful.

# Foot problems

**Bunions or hallux valgus** An inflammation or thickening of the joint of the big toe, caused by the big toe being angled excessively toward the second toe. The bunion is a symptom of the deformity and can form a sac of fluid or bursa. Often inflamed and sore, it is aggravated by tight-fitting shoes and excessive weight. A podiatrist might recommend special orthotics or shoe alterations. A bunion can be surgically removed.

**Onychomadesis** The nail lifting away from its bed is often caused by trauma, and in some cases can be caused by the nail pressing against the roof of the shoe, as in the case of athletes. The lifted nail should be clipped as short as possible to prevent it catching on anything. Wear a bandage until the nail loosens and falls off of its own accord.

**Bursitis** Usually caused by footwear rubbing the protective pad of tissue between the Achilles tendon and the heel, causing inflammation, swelling, and tenderness. Consult a doctor and change footwear.

**Athlete's foot** A fungal infection most commonly seen on the feet of athletes who spend a lot of time in locker rooms, showers, and steam rooms—the perfect environment for the infection to spread. Usually acquired by walking barefoot on infected floors. There are two varieties of athlete's foot: The first is referred to as vesicular, when the area is covered with little blisters and begins on the soles of the feet. The second, intertriginous, causes the skin between the toes to become white and saturated, splitting and peeling away to leave raw, red areas. Both varieties can be accompanied by an itchy rash. Successful treatment is possible with over-the-counter powders and lotions; the problem should clear up in a few weeks.

**Chilblains** Small, itchy, red swellings on the skin associated with cold, damp weather. As the chilblains swell and the surface of the skin cracks open, sores may develop and can become infected. This is a medical problem that needs to be treated by a doctor.

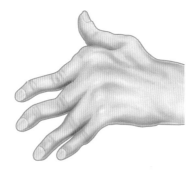

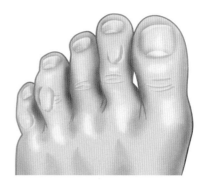

**↑ Arthritis** Affecting hands as well as feet, the synovial membranes and capsules of the joint become inflamed and swollen, with fluid retained and associated pain. Usually caused by an illness, like rheumatoid arthritis, or due to wear and tear. Avoid massage when inflammation is present. Thereafter, massage will help eliminate fluid buildup and will help keep the joints mobile. Medical attention is needed.

**↑ Corns** A buildup of dead skin in a small area as a result of pressure and friction. Unlike calluses, however, corns are usually found over a bony protuberance, such as a joint or bone. The buildup of hard skin is usually cone-shaped with the pointed part, the nucleus, facing inwards. When this nucleus presses onto a nerve, it causes pain. The various types of corns include hard corns, soft corns, seed corns, vascular and neuro-vascular corns, and fibrous corns.

**Hammer toes** A condition where one or more of the toes becomes permanently humped and flexed. Caused by ill-fitting shoes, this will need a chiropodist's consultation.

**Callus** Thickened or raised layers of hard, dead skin that form from repeated friction and pressure where your feet rub against your shoes. Calluses can become painful if allowed to grow too thick, so use a pumice stone or chiropody sponge to rub away the hard skin after you have soaked in the bath.

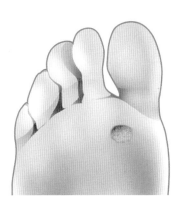

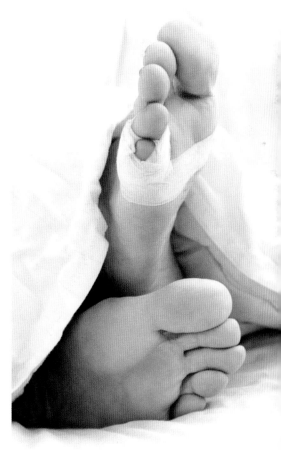

**⊕ Verrucae or verruca plantaris** These foot warts can multiply rapidly and grow larger if not treated immediately. Caused by a viral infection, verrucae resemble corns but are usually moist and have a black speck in their center. Because they are highly infectious, standard disinfection procedures are not sufficient to prevent their transmission; sterilization will be needed and you must discard all items that have been in contact with them. Consult a chiropodist.

## Did you know?

Our feet contain around 250,000 sweat glands, and they perspire more than any other part of the body. On average, each foot produces a glass of sweat each day!

# Chapter 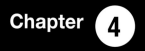 4

# TIPS, WRAPS, ACRYLICS, AND GELS

There are three main overlay systems—acrylic or liquid and powder, UV gel, and fiberglass. The acrylic system uses a liquid and powder that, when mixed together, form a solid. It is considered to be the strongest, most durable system and probably the most popular. The UV gel system is a "pre-mixed" product that forms a solid when exposed to ultraviolet (UV) light; it is a very easy, low-odor system. Fiberglass is a system that uses a fiber mesh, which can be manmade fiberglass or a natural silk or cotton, along with a resin that hardens.

When choosing a method to work with, it boils down to preferences, although it would be sensible to master one system first before moving on to any of the others. Most technicians tend to favor one method over the others, but it is best to investigate the merits of each system, consider their advantages and disadvantages and the tools and equipment you'd need, and then invest in one system with a second as a backup.

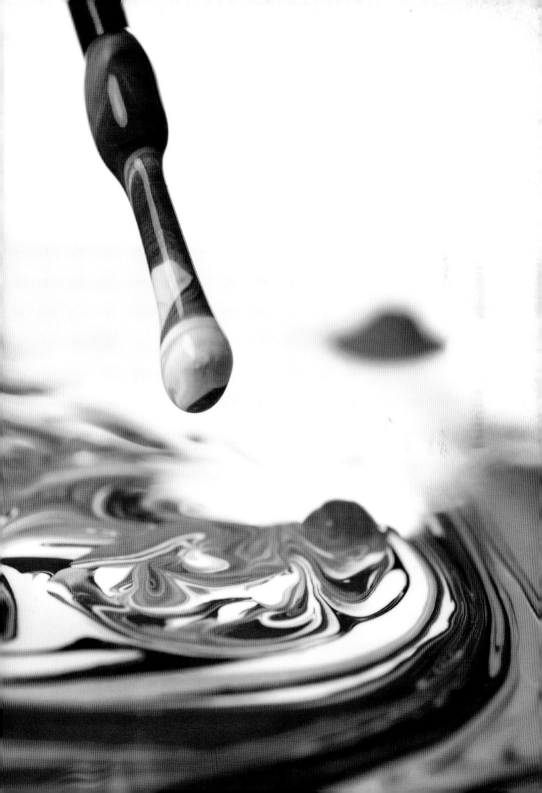

# PREPARING THE NAIL PLATE

Before applying nail enhancements, the natural nail needs to be prepared, making sure it's clean and free from nonliving tissue to enable the product to adhere effectively. This process shouldn't be rushed—taking extra care at this stage will save you considerable time later on, and more importantly, will avoid problems that could damage the natural nail. No matter what system you choose to work with, the natural nail should be prepared in the same way.

## ➲ step 1

Sanitization is the first step to ensure your hands are clean. If soap and water are used, take care to dry the nails and surrounding area thoroughly. Using a sanitizing gel is probably the most effective way to decontaminate the hands. By avoiding water, there is no risk of water being absorbed into the nail plate.

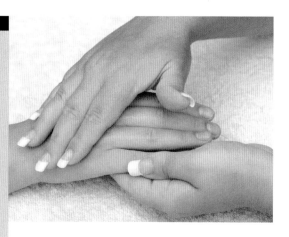

These first steps are the same for each overlay system and are repeated each time.

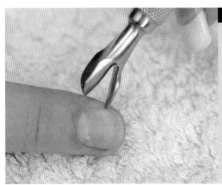

**⊖ step 2**

Removing the true cuticle is essential to ensure any overlay products bond properly; if they do not, the product will lift. Hold a cuticle knife flat on the nail plate and scrape toward the nail fold. If the tool is held upright, you can dig into the nail plate and damage the nail. Any hangnails should also be removed at this stage. Paying particular attention to the cuticle and sidewall areas, gently lift the nail folds.

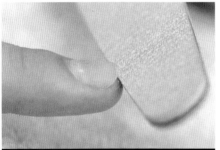

**⬆ step 3**

Remove the nail plate's shine with either a white block or a 200-grit file in the direction of the nail growth. File and bevel the nail to a 45° angle so the free edge can be filed to fit into the nail tip.

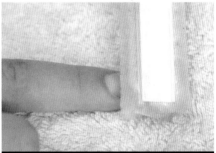

**⬆ step 4**

Use a nonstatic brush to remove dust before applying the dehydrator.

**➔ step 5**

Cleanse the nail plate with pH balancer, dehydrator, or acetone-free varnish remover, to remove dust and oils. This will also ensure that no bacteria is trapped between the natural nail and the overlay, and will dehydrate the nail plate, making it more receptive to acrylic. The nail plate is porous and needs to dry and shrink back to its original size and shape prior to applying an overlay.

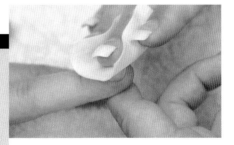

**step 6**

Continue to the next stage of your chosen system.

# LIQUID AND POWDER SYSTEM

Acrylic (sculptured) nails are strong, natural-looking, and durable, and with the development of new products, they are simple and quick to achieve. The liquid and powder system is one of the hardest systems to apply, but once mastered, its versatility is immense. This pliable product can be sculpted onto a tip, or a free-form; it can be used to correct difficult nails shapes and to reinforce weak nails.

## Sculptured acrylic

Acrylic is produced from the combination of a liquid monomer and a polymer powder, and this mixing together results in several stages. The first stage is when the monomer reacts with the powder; additives are released and a "swelling" or "melting" occurs. Then, the polymerization takes place and the product is more gel-like and easy to move around. The final curing takes place usually within 3 to 10 minutes, when the overlay becomes hard enough to file (or makes a clicking sound when tapped). This process will continue for a few hours—be careful of hard knocks as they can interfere with and damage the artificial nail.

Once the product has been applied, it hardens, polymerizes, or cures with the warmth of the environment and the temperature of the nail. Crystallization may occur if the liquid and powder is subjected to cold environments, or when applied to nails that are cold. Most liquid monomers have added stabilizers to prevent crystallization, or a separate product called a "monomer enhancer" that you can add to your dappen dish prior to application.

Most liquid and powder systems are not completely compatible with the nail plate; they will need an application of primer to increase adhesion. Primer helps prepare the surface by burning off the bacteria and oils; it will also dehydrate the nail plate and create a more receptive surface for the acrylic to adhere to. The nail plate is porous and acid-based primers can be corrosive to the underlying tissues of the nail bed. One thin coat of primer, prior to acrylic application, is all that is needed. If you are finding the need to over-flood the nail plate with primer, or you find you need two coats to produce an adequate bond, there is something wrong. You may find you'll have to look at either the product you are using or changing your application technique.

### Materials

In addition to an appropriate manicure workstation or equivalent, you will need the following: three dappen dishes; sable applicator brush; a cuticle stick; primer or acrylic bonding agent; sanitizing solution; acrylic powder in clear, white, and pink; acrylic liquid; manufacturer's instructions; nail forms; files and buffers; base coat, top coat, and chosen nail varnish.

## step 1

Prepare the nail by carefully removing all traces of cuticle from the nail plate and then dehydrating. See page 121.

## step 2

Buff the natural nail surface and file free edge to shape.

## step 3

Apply one coat of acrylic bonding agent or primer to the natural nail to help bond the keratin with the polymer.

## ⬇ step 4

Attach the chosen form to the finger, ensuring that it fits correctly. Hold the form securely in position during application. If you are using a reusable form, slide it onto the finger, making sure the free edge of the nail fits over it and sits snugly. If disposable forms are used, peel one from its paper backing, then bend into an arch to fit the natural nail shape, slide onto the finger, and press the adhesive backing to the sides of the finger. Check to see that the form is fitting securely under the free edge and sits level with the natural nail.

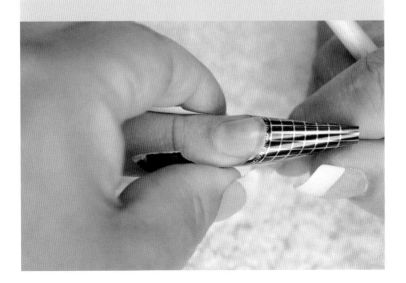

### ➔ step 5

Pour acrylic liquid (monomer) and acrylic powder (polymer) into separate glass containers or dappen dishes. (If you are using the two-color method, you'll need three containers—one for the white tip powder; one for the clear, natural, or pink powder; and one for the acrylic liquid, which is three-quarters full.) Dip the brush into the liquid, submerging the bristles into the liquid to rid it of air pockets and then press against the dish to release any excess. Wipe the brush carefully on a paper towel.

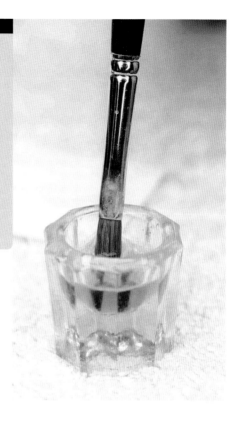

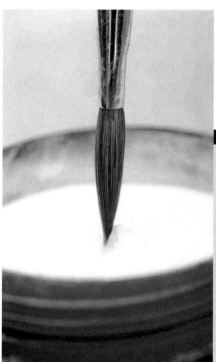

### ➔ step 6

Dip the tip of the brush gently into the white powder, sweeping the brush across the surface, slightly rotating, until it has gathered as much powder as the brush can hold and is large enough to shape the entire free edge extension. Count to three slowly, to allow the liquid in the brush to make contact with the powder, before removing the brush from the second container.

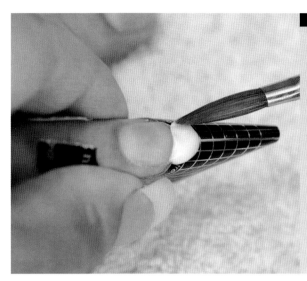

### ⊖ step 7

Place the resulting acrylic ball on the center of the nail form where it joins the free edge at the smile line. Allow the bead to settle prior to manipulation. Wait a few seconds, then gently pat, press, and dab to shape using the middle portion of the brush. Wipe the brush gently on the paper towel to remove any excess product from the brush.

### ➋ step 8

Keep the sides parallel and shape continuously along the free edge. Dabbing creates a more natural-looking nail. If the two-color acrylic method is used, the natural free edge line must be followed with the white powder to create the French manicure look.

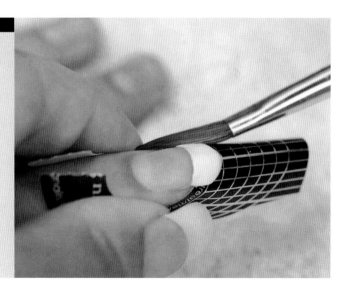

### step 9

Create a second ball of acrylic using the pink acrylic powder.

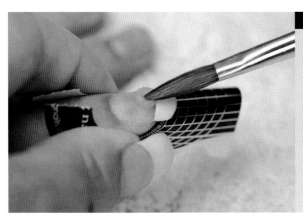

### ← step 10

Place the second ball of acrylic on the natural nail next to the free edge line in the center of the nail.

### step 11

Shape the ball by dabbing and pressing out to the side walls, making sure the product is very thin around all edges.

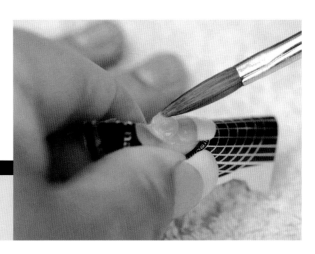

### → step 12

Place a third ball of pink acrylic at the cuticle area.

### ← step 13

Smooth the ball over the nail, gliding the brush over the nail toward the tip to remove imperfections. The edges closest to the cuticle, side wall, and free edge must be very thin to achieve the most convincing nails.

### step 14

Tap the nails with the brush handle to hear
if they make a clicking sound. This will indicate
that they are dry.

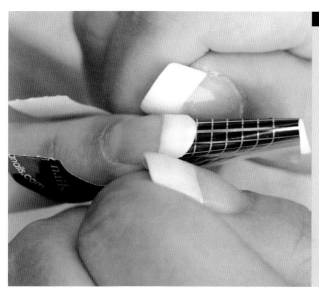

### step 15

Remove the forms once
the nails are thoroughly
dry.

### step 16

Shape the nails using a
medium-grade emery
board, then buff until the
entire surface is smooth.

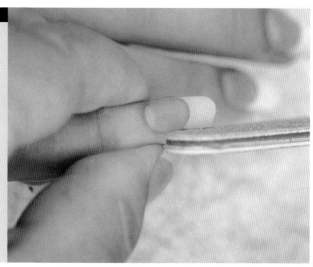

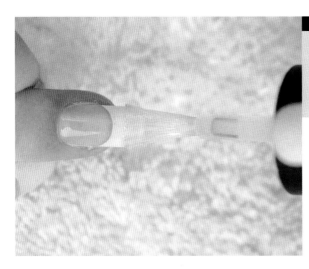

**⊖ step 17**

Finish off the nails with a layer of base coat, two coats of nail polish if desired, and a top coat. Finally, apply a drop of cuticle oil to each nail.

## Pro Tip

Finding the correct consistency is the biggest challenge for both professionals and beginners alike, especially because consistency changes from brand to brand. The correct ratio of liquid and powder is vital for strong, flexible, durable enhancements that won't lift. The opposite can result in premature lifting or even breakage. Most powder and liquid systems require a medium-wet bead, while some odorless systems may require less liquid than normal. Be sure to follow manufacturer's instructions, as consistency and ratio mix will differ from brand to brand. Never mix brands—such as a liquid monomer from one brand and a powder from another—because the catalyst system might not be compatible and other additives might not work together. Always use a system that is designed to be used together.

**Too dry** Will result in unsightly, thick nails, premature lifting, and nails that are prone to breakages.

**Too wet** Will cause lifting. While a wet bead may assist in creating a flawless finish and less filing, it can result in an overlay that is prone to lifting and flaking.

**Medium-wet** Will produce a strong, flexible, yet durable enhancement.

**Method:** Place the bead onto the tip. Do not move or touch it with your brush and wait for 5–7 seconds. If the bead reduces by half in height and runs, almost doubling in diameter, it is too wet. If the bead looks slightly cloudy and stays virtually the same height and shape, it is too dry. A medium-wet bead will only lose about 25 percent of its height and increase in diameter by about 25 percent. Don't brush your acrylic on—use gentle yet firm patting and gliding motions.

# Acrylic overlay

A thin layer of acrylic coating is laid over the natural nail, or over tips, to reinforce and strengthen them.

**step 1**

Prepare the nail by carefully removing all traces of cuticle from the nail plate and then dehydrating. See page 121.

**step 2**

Buff the natural nail surfaces and free edges to shape. See page 121. Apply a drop of nail adhesive to the nail tip, which needs to be held at a 45° angle. Place the top of the tip at the free edge, roll back, press down, and hold in place.

**step 3**

Trim the tips with a special nail trimmer.

**step 4**

Shape the tips away with a nail file and smooth away any rough edges.

**step 5**

Blend the tip seam where it joins the nail and shape the free edge with a medium to fine file.

**step 6**

Buff the nails, blending and smoothing carefully; once the dust is removed, the nails should be clean and oil-free.

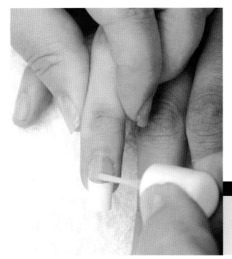

These first steps are the same for each overlay system and are repeated each time.

**◉ step 7**

Apply one coat of acrylic bonding agent or primer to the natural nail to help to bond the keratin with the polymer.

### ➔ step 8

The best way to apply acrylic is with the ball method: Dip the brush into the liquid and press against the dish to release any excess. Sweep the tip of the brush across the surface of the powder until it has gathered as much powder as it can hold and is large enough to cover the entire nail. Apply the ball of product to the center of the nail.

French manicure effect: If a white tip is required, then start by applying a white sculpting gel to the free edge of the tip or nail, working it into a smile line, following the smile line of the natural nail. Then apply a clear bead to the stress line, drawing it down to meet the white smile line, and fill.

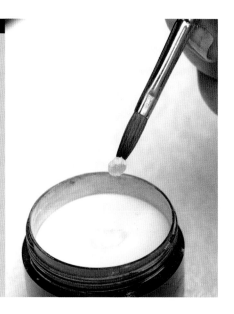

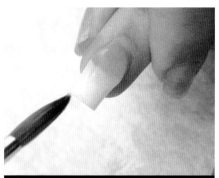

### ↑ step 9

Working quickly while it is still wet, push the acrylic back to fill the sides and complete the nail overlay. Curing times vary, so check your manufacturer's instructions before filing and buffing.

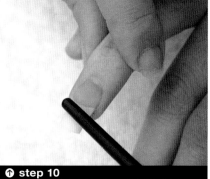

### ↑ step 10

Tap the nails and listen for the clicking sound that indicates when the product has completely cured. File and buff the nails, then complete according to your needs—with base coat, polish, and top coat. Apply a drop of cuticle oil to each cuticle.

# Acrylic nail fill-ins and maintenance

Fills are essential every two weeks to maintain acrylic nails.

- Remove nail polish with acetone-free polish remover and check each nail for lifting, cracks, chips, infections, or damage to the cuticle and surrounds.
- Push back and neaten cuticles, removing any lifted acrylic by clipping it away with acrylic nippers. Protective eyewear is recommended at this stage, as pieces can fly all over the place.
- Scrub and sanitize, then file down to your required length, straighten sidewalls, and buff the regrowth area to remove shine.
- Remove any dust, apply sanitizer to regrowth area, and dry thoroughly.
- If replacing a white French manicure overlay, you need to remove most of the last application. If not, just thin down and remove the bulk— remembering that the stress area has moved forward slightly.
- Carefully buff close to the cuticle area to smooth out the seam where the natural nail has grown

through. Any lifting will need to be corrected and any buffing must be done with the utmost care to avoid damaging the natural nail.

- Remove dust and apply dehydrator to cleanse the regrowth area.
- If you are backfilling, or redefining the French manicure smile line, apply a small bead of white product to the free edge and redefine the smile line, making sure you push product into the corners of the sidewall.
- Place a small bead in the center, push to the sidewalls and then toward the cuticle area.
- If you are not backfilling, place a small bead in the center of the nail and press to the sidewalls, also pressing a thin layer out to the free edge. Place a second bead in the center, just below this, and push over toward the cuticle, making sure to push product down at the cuticle to help prevent lifting.
- File and buff, then wash to remove excess oil, and polish if desired.
- To rebalance, you will need to remove the apex that has grown forward to the wrong place, and replace it in the correct position. Fill the regrowth area and put the smile line back where it should be.

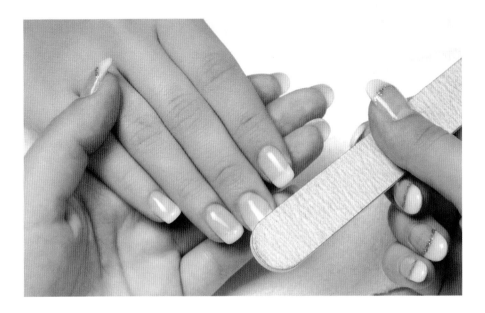

# UV GEL SYSTEM

The UV gel system is a pre-mixed system of application for which the only other equipment needed is the UV light source. The big advantage of this system is that it is virtually odor-free and there is no mixing or worrying about mix ratios and consistency. UV light must penetrate completely through the gel for it to polymerize or cure all oligomers properly. As with all the systems, there are many application techniques specific to individual companies and you'd need to be versed in their specific formulations before working with their products. Some companies will have just one gel, while others have a three-phase system which includes a builder gel, a base gel, and a top coat gel.

All gels belong to the acrylic family and are based on the methacrylate and acrylate families. Made from oligomers, which are the short pre-joined chains of molecules (neither monomer nor polymer), they have a thicker consistency, resulting in lower evaporation and odor levels. Advantages of this system are its ease of application and the fact that it is a low-odor system. Also, the smooth finish of the gel means less buffing and filing to finish off. A disadvantage with some of these systems is the long curing times between layers.

## Materials

You will need sanitizer, assorted nail tips if the product is not being sculpted, adhesive, files and buffers, cuticle conditioner, primer, gels—usually three, depending on the system: foundation gel, builder gel, and sealer gel (other systems might use one gel for all layers)—plus three gel brushes, one for each gel; a curing UV lamp; gel remover; and a brush cleaner.

**step 1**

Prepare the nail by carefully removing all traces of cuticle from the nail plate and then dehydrating. See page 121.

**step 2**

Buff the natural nail surfaces and free edges and file to shape. Add a drop of nail adhesive to the nail tip, which should be held at a 45° angle. Place the top of the tip at the free edge, roll back, press down, and hold in place.

## step 3

Trim the tips with a special nail-tip edge trimmer.

## step 4

Shape the tips with a nail file and smooth any rough edges away.

## step 5

Blend the tip seam where it joins the nail and shape the free edge with a medium to fine file.

## step 6

Buff the nails and smooth carefully.

These first steps are the same for each overlay system and are repeated each time.

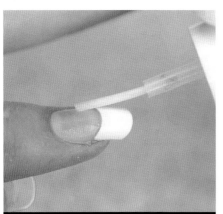

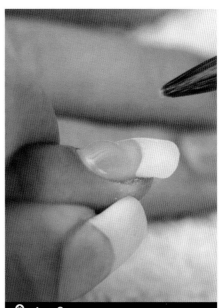

## ⬆ step 7

Depending on whether the products being applied need a primer, apply primer to the whole nail. Then apply a coat of foundation gel or bonder to the whole nail, making sure you leave a small margin around the cuticle and sidewalls (this will apply to each layer) and set it under the light.

## ⬆ step 8

With the sticky residue on the surface, apply a layer of builder gel, sculpture gel, or bonder to the whole nail. Cure under the lamp, making sure each finger is correctly placed and exposed to the UV light—development time will vary depending on which brand you are working with.

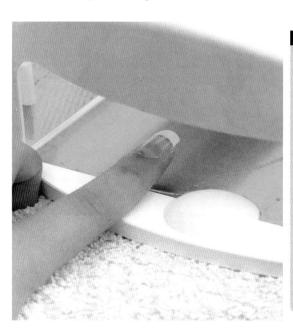

### ← step 9

Apply a coat of sealant gel and cure with the lamp, making sure each finger is correctly placed and exposed to the UV light—development time will vary depending on the brand you are working with.

### → step 10

You may need to wipe residue or small imperfections from the surface of the nail with the appropriate cleanser, like acetone, before buffing. Shape nails with a high-grit file, buff to a natural shine, or apply a thin layer of gel. Cure to produce a high gloss after the sticky layer is removed. If you go with the second option, all the dust created from the buffing must be carefully removed with a finishing wipe on a tissue and the paper towel carefully removed with all the dust that has collected before you apply the gel.

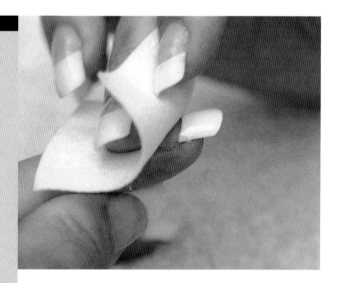

### step 11

Apply oil and massage.

# FIBERGLASS SYSTEM

Fiber wraps are perfect for reinforcing and strengthening weaker nails and are useful for patching and repairing broken ones. This method involves the application of a fiber mesh, usually silk or fiberglass, but sometimes cotton or linen—natural fibers tend to soak up the resin, while fiberglass retains its integrity and adds flexibility and strength to the resin.

## Fiber wraps

The resin used with fiberglass is cryanoacrylate; this encases the fabric mesh and has little strength without it. Fiberglass fabrics can be clear, white, or pink, and are sold in strips or a dispensing box. The resin is cured or dried by an activator, which speeds up the drying time. This is also a system that is quick to remove, with little to no damage to the natural nail. It is ideal as a natural nail repair, and it is also a low-odor option if using a paint-on activator. However, the overlay is quite thin and not as strong as the structured nail in other systems. There are numerous suppliers and you will need to experiment before investing in any wrap system.

### Materials

You will need the following: sanitizing solution, tips, adhesive, nail preparation products, fiberglass or silk, sharp small scissors, resin (brush-on or nozzle and applicator), activator or accelerator (spray or brush-on), manufacturer's instructions, files and buffers, and nail polish (if you intend to paint the nails).

### step 1

Prepare the nail by carefully removing all traces of cuticle from the nail plate and then dehydrating. See page 121.

### step 2

Buff natural nail surfaces and file free edges to shape. Apply a drop of nail adhesive to the nail tip, which should be held at a 45° angle. Place the top of the tip at the free edge, roll back, press down, and hold in place.

### step 3

Trim the tips with a special nail trimmer.

### step 4

Shape the tips with a nail file and smooth rough edges away.

### step 5

Blend the tip seam where it joins the nail and shape the free edge with a medium to fine file.

### step 6

Carefully buff and smooth the nails.

These first steps are the same for each overlay system and are repeated each time.

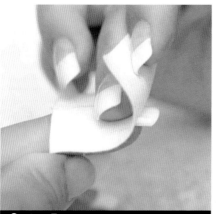

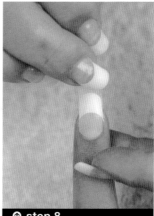

### ⬆ step 7

Ensure the nails with tips are clean and dehydrated; this system does not need priming, because the buffed surfaces are enough to hold the overlay.

### ⬆ step 8

Apply the self-adhesive microfiber wrap, trim the sides if needed, and cut the fabric slightly shorter than the tip to allow the tip to be sealed with resin.

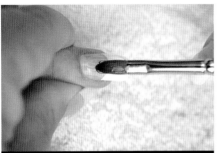

**⊕ step 9**

Apply one or two coats of thin acrylic resin, being careful not to touch the skin. Leave a tiny margin of bare nail around the edges to ensure proper adhesion.

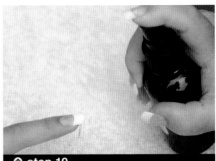

**⊕ step 10**

If spray activator is being used, don't spray too closely, as pitting of the resin may occur; only minute amounts are needed—too much can result in a heat reaction that may be uncomfortable. If using the brush, spread the resin with the activator brush while keeping the product off the skin. The brushes can get blocked up with polymerized resin and will need to be placed in a solvent between uses to keep them clean.

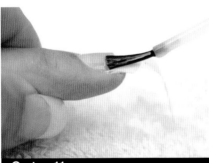

**⊕ step 11**

Repeat resin and activator for another layer if more strength is required.

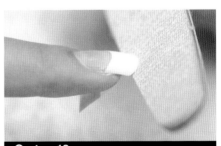

**⊕ step 12**

When dry, the remnants of the fiber wraps are cut away. Buff any roughness until smooth. If silk or fiberglass fabric has been used, nail polish is optional, as the nail looks completely natural.

**step 13**

Finally remove all dust and apply oil to the nail surface, cuticle, and surrounding skin to eliminate dryness. Wipe over with non-acetone nail varnish and apply nail polish as required.

# CHOOSING THE RIGHT TIP

Most tips have a full contact area, but you will need to remove most of it before applying it to the natural nail; full contact areas are more prone to air pockets because of the larger surface. The newest tips have a reduced contact area, called a speed well or quarter well, and are known as express tips. Designed with no stopping point, which allows you to place the tip anywhere on the nails, they are quicker to attach, more efficient, and require less filing.

## Getting it right

- Pre-tailor the tip before application, making sure you follow the manufacturer's application instructions, as techniques vary hugely from brand to brand. Bear in mind that this book is a guide and methods may vary.
- Size tips—to ensure a perfect fit with the natural nail's free edge and matching the ridge in the well of the tip. Check if the nail fits into the grooves on either side of the natural nail. If it doesn't fit, lifting and cracking of the nail could result in damage to the nail plate.
- Always pre-tailor to suit the natural nail shape, shaping the tip to fit before applying; it cannot be changed once it is on the finger.
- When applying a tip with full contact area, be

careful to avoid getting bubbles under the tip—the bubbles will be visible and provide areas for bacteria and fungus to thrive.
- A full contact area needs careful blending to avoid a visible shadow showing through the overlay; it will not look as defined and clear as a smaller contact area (tips should not cover more than 30 percent of the natural nail).
- To minimize the contact area, cut out a "v" shape with scissors or clippers, or file at the correct angle to create a curved edge, which will ensure extra protection and support at the sidewalls of the free edge of the natural nail.
- With a minimal contact area, it is easier to place the tip at the right angle, resulting in the most natural-looking nail and the least damage to the natural nail.

- Apply a small amount of adhesive to the well of the nail. This will prevent it from seeping down the sidewalls and prepare and soften the plastic for accurate placement.
- Press the tip onto the natural nail, holding the tip at a 45° angle, then lever into place, making sure the well of the tip is butting into the natural nail's free edge. Ensure there are no bubbles and apply pressure.
- Excess adhesive must be removed from under the free edge, the nail plate, and surrounding tissue before it dries.
- Cut the tip to the desired length with tip cutters, by angling the cutter under the hand. A slightly curved oval shape will result; the more upright the angle of the cutter, the straighter the edge.
- Shape the free edge to the required shape and length, then taper and blend the sidewalls of the natural nail.
- Buff the ledge level with the natural nail, being careful not to file the natural nail. Thin the entire tip, thinning out the free edge until it appears translucent. Then, carefully avoiding working in one area to prevent heat buildup, refine zone 2 (the stress area). Do this until there is no shadow and the tip area is transparent and thin, ensuring the smile line is refined. Check the arch is even and the lower arch is correct. The tips are now the ideal canvas onto which the overlay can be applied.

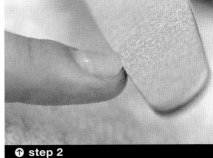

**⬆ step 2**

File and bevel the nail to a 45° angle.

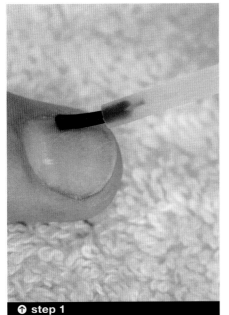

**⬆ step 1**

Apply pH balancer to entire nail plate.

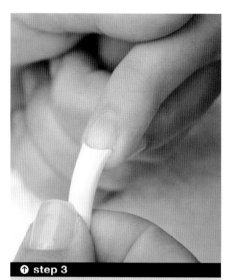

**⬆ step 3**

Size, pre-fit, and tailor the tips to suit your natural nail shape.

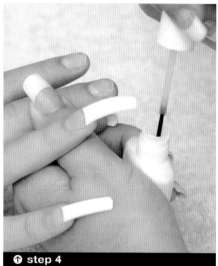

**⬆ step 4**

Apply a small amount of adhesive to the tip of the natural nail.

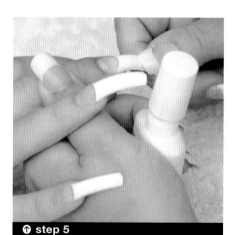

**⬆ step 5**

Press tip onto natural nail tip, holding at a 45° angle to ensure there are no air bubbles.

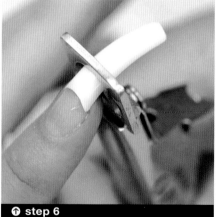

**⬆ step 6**

Cut the tips to the desired length using clippers—the angle of the clipper blade will determine the outline of the finished shape—oval, square, or tapered. If the clipper is angled under your hand, a slightly oval shape will result. The more upright the clipper, the straighter the edge.

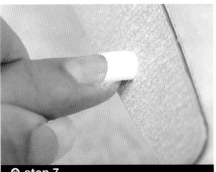

### ⬆ step 7

File the tips to the desired shape and remove any debris that may have collected underneath during filing.

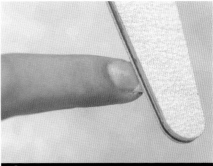

### ⬆ step 8

Blend the tips with the natural nail with a 240-grit buffer, making sure the seam is flush with the natural nail. Check that the upper arch is correct and even, and that the lower arch is correct. Most new tips are speed application tips with smile lines already done, which means no tip blending will be required.

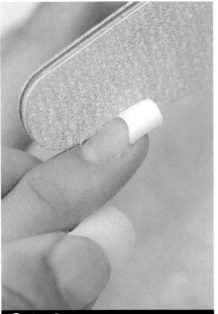

### ⬆ step 9

Define the sidewalls to blend into the sidewalls of the natural nail, and gently refine the smile line to create a natural finish.

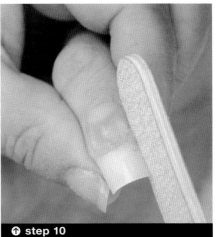

### ⬆ step 10

Check for any sharp edges before moving onto the overlay application.

# REMOVING ACRYLIC NAILS

Numerous products are available for softening, dissolving, and removing nail enhancements. Choose a removal system that is compatible or recommended by the same manufacturer as the material to be removed. Most solvents are acetone-based and will break the bonds between the polymer chains. Cyanoacrylate resin in the fiberglass system comes off the easiest, because it has the weakest bonds, making it much safer and more efficient to remove.

This is a removal method for all nail enhancements.

### ➔ step 1

Cut back the length of the nails and remove nail polish before soaking nails in a glass dish filled with about 1 inch of product remover, which is being warmed in a larger bowl of hot water. The heat accelerates the removal process by breaking down the chemical bonds.

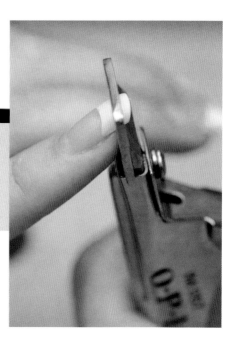

### ● step 2

Cover hands with a towel to keep the heat in and to help contain the vapors; let the hands soak for at least 20 minutes. After this time, different products will have reacted differently—some will have dissolved completely, and others will have softened and will need to be gently pried off.

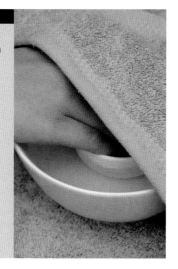

### ↑ step 3

Lift out one hand and wipe off excess fluid, then gently wipe the surface of the nails with cotton gauze wipes soaked in solvent; wipe each finger until the product has been removed.

### ● step 4

Wipe off all the nails in this way, dry them, then wash the hands to remove all traces of solvent.

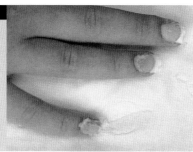

### ● step 5

Using a fine buffer, buff the surface of the natural nail to remove any last traces of product.

### step 6

Check the cuticles and reshape the free edge.

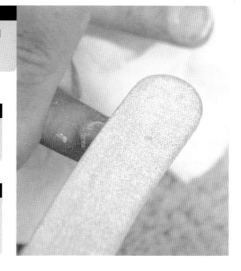

### step 7

Reapply nail extensions or rehydrate the hands with hand cream and the cuticles, sidewalls, and surrounding skin with cuticle oil.

# TROUBLESHOOTING

Being aware of all the possible contraindications or problems that could arise from wearing nail extensions is imperative, as it will allow you to deal with them effectively if and when they occur. Signs to look for include: separation of the hyponychium, sensitivity and discomfort when pressure is applied to the nail bed, or separation of the nail plate from the nail bed. If any of these signs are discovered, the product will have to be removed and its use discontinued—any separation of the nail plate from the nail bed will need to be treated by a medical practitioner.

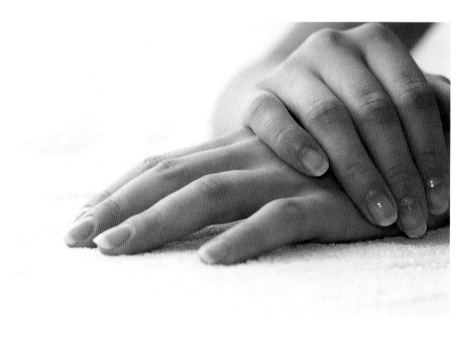

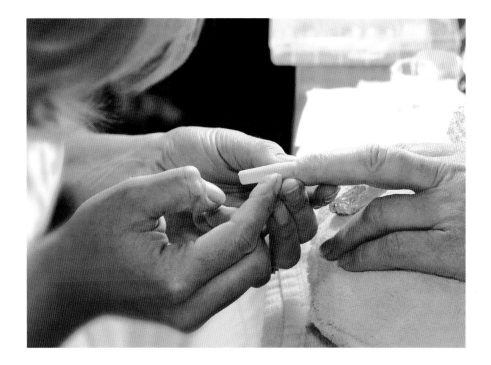

## Allergies

Alleries will, in all likelihood, result in a reaction to some of the product used in nail extensions. If there is any risk of an allergic reaction, it is best to do a patch test, allowing 24 hours for a response. Any redness or inflammation would indicate an adverse reaction, in which case you should discontinue usage immediately.

## Patch testing

To do a patch test, apply the nail liquid or gel to a bandage, and stick it onto the inside of your elbow for 24 hours. Additionally, you could also trial-fit one nail and then wait for 48 hours to check that there is no adverse reaction to the product before completing a full set. If there is any doubt about a condition, do not continue—seek specialist advice.

## Nail porosity

The nail plate is porous and will absorb moisture and oil, swelling imperceptibly in the process. Once it dries out again, it shrinks back to its original state. This is why using any oils or soaking

methods before fitting nail extensions will cause lifting of the product. To ensure adequate adhesion, the nail must be oil- and moisture-free, and a dehydrator, or acetone, should be applied before any technique is started. The dehydrator also serves as a sanitizer, eliminating any likelihood of bacteria.

## Lifting

The natural nail plate is flexible, particularly around the cuticle, so too much pressure will make it bend. The artificial nail product is not flexible, and placing too much direct pressure in a thin area will cause it to flex and break its adhesion, resulting in lifting. Lifting is also caused by excessive pressure when surface filing, improper preparation of the nail plate prior to treatment, too much pressure when pushing cuticles back for nail-fill treatment, or an incorrect mix ratio.

# BROKEN NAIL EMERGENCY

The first thing to do with a broken nail is to secure it, to prevent further damage until you can get home or to a nail salon.

## DIY advice

If the nail is torn but not completely broken off while you are away from home, try wrapping the fingertip with adhesive tape or a bandage, first up and over the tip and then around the nail. Make sure you keep a bit of slack inside so the nail is not bent. Band-Aids especially designed for fingertips work best. If you use tape, first protect the nail surface with a bit of tissue to prevent the tape from sticking to the nail. An added benefit of covering the fingertip is that you will naturally avoid using that finger, thus minimizing further trauma.

Once you get home, use a small pair of scissors to gently cut away the tape—now you can assess the damage. Do not pick at the nail. If it is just a slight tear on the side, you may get by simply by using extra coats of a nail strengthener containing nylon fibers. It may also be a good idea to slightly shorten the nail so it will be less likely to bang into

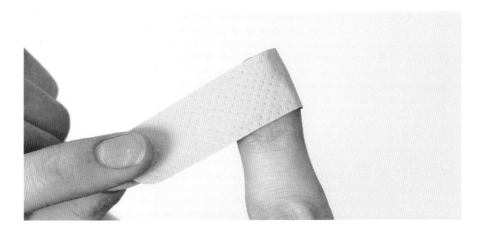

things, causing more damage. If the nail is completely off, or torn more than one-quarter of the width of the nail, you must take more serious measures. Keep on hand an emergency nail repair kit containing both powdered and liquid acrylic, as well as a circular nail buffer. If a nail breaks, accept that it will never be as good as new until it grows back naturally. The easier approach is just to accept the loss and trim the others down a bit so that the broken nail does not look so awkward while it grows back.

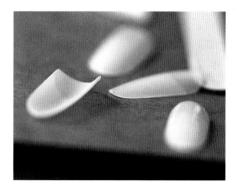

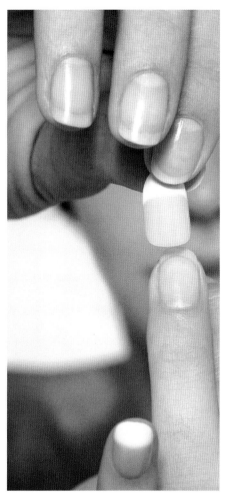

- Clean the nail with soap, then rinse it with water and allow to dry.
- Apply the acrylic in a thick coat that covers the nail. Let this dry completely. Carefully buff the nail down to a smooth surface that forms a "cap" over the broken nail. Keep the nail as short as possible; the longer the nail, the more you will bang it.
- Apply a second coat and buff down again. Some kits come with a thin silk or nylon sheet to be placed between coats for added strength. Take your time to create a realistic cap over the nail.
- Once dried, apply a coat of hardener, with nylon fibers, daily. When the natural nail has grown long enough, remove the cap by soaking it in polish remover and very carefully pry it off. (Pry it a bit, then soak, then repeat as often as needed to remove it with the least damage.)
- Keep in mind that if you constantly remove the polish, you will weaken the cap with the polish remover and probably need to start the process all over again.
- As the nail grows, the base may look a bit odd as the base of the cap is exposed. You may need to remove the polish and touch up the cap a bit on the edges; it is best just to leave the cap on until it has grown enough to expose the natural nail.

**Chapter** **5**

# NAIL FASHION

Get as creative as you like; the choices are endless.
With commercially produced nail adornments from
rhinestones and gems, striping tape, appliqués, glitter,
and transfers, you really have a myriad of choices.
Nail art can be as soft and subtle or as outrageous as
your imagination allows.

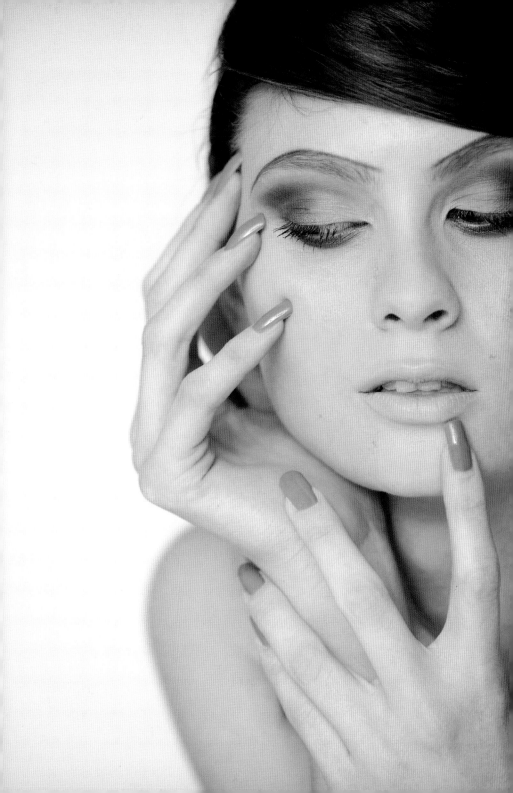

# NAIL POLISH IN FASHION

Nail polish is currently enjoying a fashion revival. Chanel's nail sensation, Rouge Noir, became the company's best-selling product ever. Its cult status rocketed when it was seen on Uma Thurman's nails in *Pulp Fiction*. Traditionally, women have always worn nail polish, but it has been gaining popularity with men as well. Special nail polish lines have been developed with unusual colors such as Testosterone (gunmetal gray), Gigolo (silver-specked black), Superman (midnight blue), and Dog (deep purple).

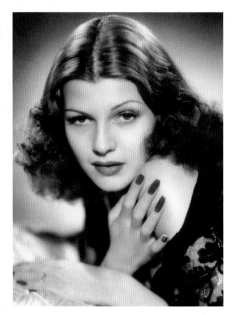

## Nail fashion of the 1940s, 1950s, and 1960s

In the 1940s there were no nail salons, as such. People would have their nails done in barber shops, and, interestingly, it was commonplace for men, as well as women, to have a manicure at the same time as having a haircut, a shave, and a shoeshine. Nonetheless, nail care was still, predominantly, a female pastime. 1940s fashion is still, today, a desirable look, as it is both classic and striking. Just think Lauren Bacall and Ava Gardner.

The 1940s saw a new trend emerge in nail fashion, due, in no small part, to the end of the Great Depression. Housewives suddenly had some spare change to spend on frivolous luxuries like manicures and cosmetics. Rita Hayworth helped advance nail fashion too, when her long, dark red, talon nails became almost as famous as she did. It became increasingly popular for women to grow their nails to extreme length, and crimson red was the color of choice. Elizabeth Arden created a color called "Schoolhouse Red," which was especially coveted, at seventy-five cents a bottle. Another change in nail fashion was shape. While nails had previously been filed into a point, the 1940s saw a more natural oval shape start to dominate nail fashion.

There were no paraffin wax manicures or aromatic salt rubs in the 1940s, no fiberglass or silk wraps either. It might seem odd to the modern woman, but in the 1940s, tea bags, coffee filters, and household cement were used as treatments instead. Bizarrely, cigarette papers, perm papers, and airplane glue were also sometimes used for wraps! Another nail fashion of the 1940s was bleaching the tips of one's nails with a white nail pencil. This technique is still sometimes used today.

After the end of WWII, in 1945, fashion saw a gradual escalation of unrestricted creativity. In 1947, Christian Dior's "New Look" changed the face of fashion forever. Femininity was exaggerated, but so was feminism, though some remnants of wartime fashions still remained. When the Cold War began, mid-decade, rations were brought back to the American people, and women went back to the workplace. This had a profound effect on fashion and nail fashion.

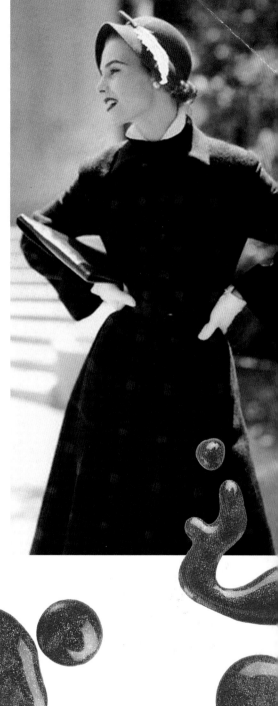

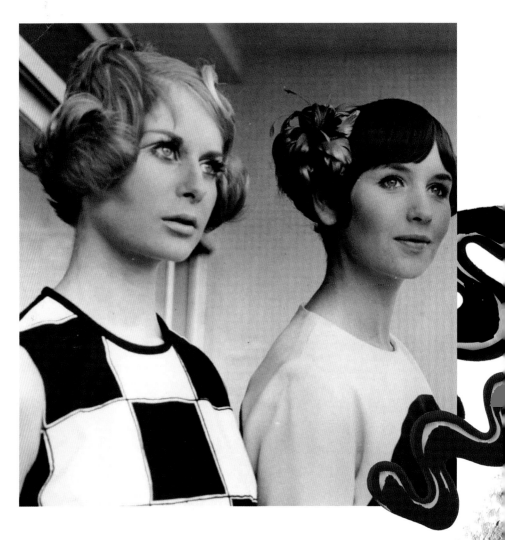

By the 1950s, dark reds were out. It became very fashionable to emphasize one's eyes more strongly, with perhaps less attention being paid to lips and nails. Titanium was added to tone down the brightness of products, providing a shimmering gleam. Frosted nail polishes in pink, peach, silver, and a host of other colors began to appear, although matte red was still very popular. Another trend specific to the 1950s was to cover only the top third of the nail in a wrap. This was referred to as a Juliette manicure. In 1957, Thomas Slack issued a patent for a "platform" that was fitted around the nail edge, designed to help manicurists apply extensions to the natural nail. Made of foil, it was used to apply the first acrylic nails, called Pattinail.

In the late 1950s, Max Factor brought out a lipstick color called "Strawberry Meringue," which was a pastel pearly pink and matched the softer shades of nail polishes around at the time. As the 1950s ended, *Vogue* magazine started to coordinate the colors of the season's latest clothes with those of cosmetics. Eventually all the makeup houses followed, producing ranges that picked up color changes. The 1960s produced some very eclectic styles and trends.

The 1960s saw London at the forefront of fashion for the first time. Mary Quant introduced the miniskirt to the mass population, while shops like Snob, Biba, and Mr. Freedom were also pushing the boundaries of acceptable fashion. Black and white was "in" again, and white lipstick became popular, along with black nail polish. In contrast, feminism became a big deal in the 1960s, and the shorter length that was fashionable for women to wear their nails reflects this. Shorter nails were also more practical, since so many more women had begun professional careers. Being sophisticated was just as cool as being a free-spirited hippy in the 1960s, despite what many young people of today might think.

In terms of nail color, the 1960s were incredibly diverse. Purple was always popular, but so were green, yellow, orange, and even brown. In many cities across the world, the 1960s were years of individualism, expressionism, and especially, continued innovation. For example, nail art was born in the form of pop art nail transfers, which were created in the vein of Andy Warhol. However, since there was still a strong cosmetic trend to emphasize the eyes, perpetuated by the dramatic makeup worn by Warhol's muse, Edie Sedgwick, red lips and nails were less frequently seen.

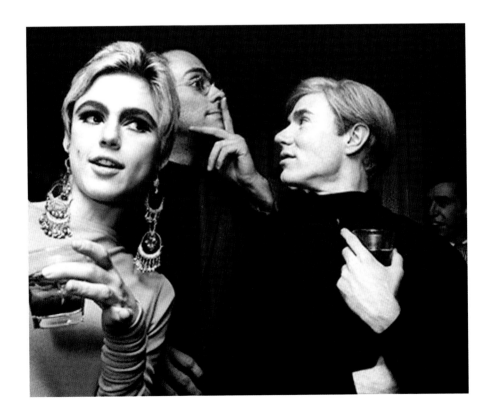

Today, traditional colors for nail polish are red, all types of pink, and flesh-colored shades, although more unusual shades are also available, such as yellow, orange, black, and even green. French manicures mimic the colors of natural nails, with flesh tones being painted on the nail and white on the tips. Nail polish can be found in nearly every color and shade imaginable. Black or other very dark nail polish has been popular among goths and punks, but it has now gained popularity in the mainstream fashion world too. Nail polish may also be used to complete an outfit and is often chosen to match the colors of one's clothing.

Colors with glitter and metallic sheens are popular with teens, while clear and pink remain all-time favorites. Designs are painted on one nail, usually the ring finger, with thinner nail brushes. Designs include flowers, strokes of lines, and even more detailed designs applied with airbrush tools, usually on acrylic nails.

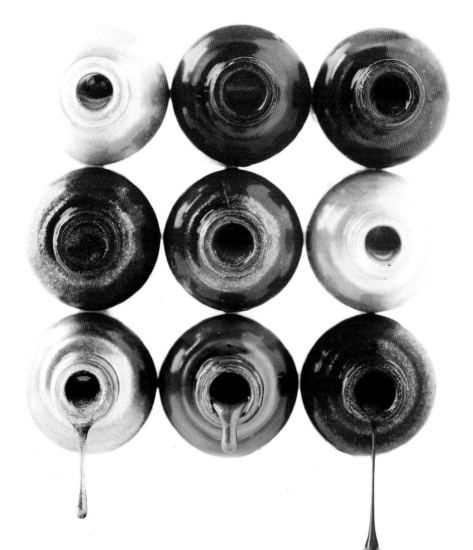

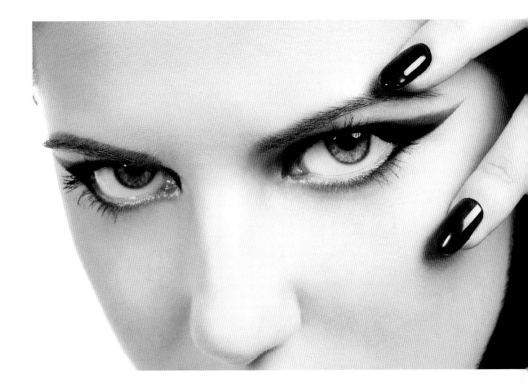

## Polish application styles

1 **Full coverage**—for expert coverage, dip the brush and then circle the inside of the bottleneck with the brush to remove any excess polish. Apply the polish with the drip on the underside of the brush. Place the polish two-thirds of the way down the nail plate and press the polish toward the cuticle area. Then brush down the nail using soft strokes; the average nail takes three or four strokes for full coverage. Clean up around the nails with a cuticle stick dipped in acetone, or use a polish corrector pen.

2 **Free edge**—the free edge of the nail is unpolished to help keep the nail polish from chipping. The result looks much like a reversed French manicure.

3 **Hairline tip**—the nail plate is polished and a millimeter of polish is removed from the free edge to prevent chipping.

4 **Slim line or free walls**—leave a narrow margin on each side of the nail plate, to make a wide nail appear longer and more elegant.

5 **Half-moon or lunula**—the half-moon or "lunula" at the base of the nail is left free of polish. This is difficult to do and requires practice.

# INTRODUCING NAIL ART

It is one thing to have perfectly manicured nails, but it is something else entirely to actually wear a piece of art on your nails. If you want to make a real fashion statement, if you're bored with solid colors and simple French manicures, nail art really is the answer. In our acutely fashion-conscious modern world, it is no surprise that nail art is growing increasingly popular with young women across the globe. Nail art is less traditional, more unique, and completely accessible. It must be said, however, that nail art requires skill and patience to master, as there are so many different techniques and materials that can be used.

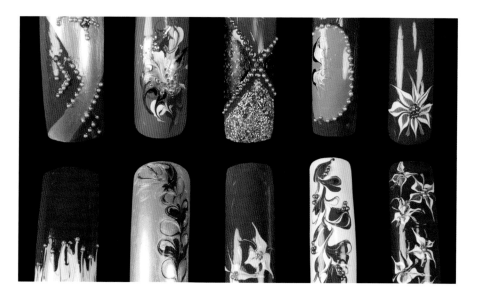

French nail art, in particular, is very much in vogue at the moment. Perhaps this is because the ever-popular, but more conventional, French manicure provides a perfect canvas for creativity, since the majority of the nail is colorless. Nail art is extremely popular among designers showing collections on the catwalk, because it is such an expressive way of complementing clothes and personal style.

Permanent nail art designs can be created with the help of dried flowers, glitters, acrylic shapes, rhinestones, and bullion beads, although there are new innovations all the time. The process for embedding is very simple; however if you aren't feeling confident of trying it yourself, almost all nail salons now employ professionals who can do the job perfectly for you.

Airbrush designs are another good way to add art to your nails. This requires a machine with a stencil to spray paint the design onto your nail. However, since the machine needed is rather expensive, it's best to get this done by a professional too. Airbrush designs are not as popular as hand-painted patterns though—they are not nearly as individual!

The hand-painted pattern is probably the most popular form of nail art. Jungle and animal themes are especially trendy, although niche designs are becoming more desirable, like seasonal images for Christmas or Halloween. The easiest way to draw onto your nails is to cut a toothpick in half and then dip the newly blunt end into the nail polish you want to use for the design. Make five tiny dots in a circle, forming a flower. Then add glitter or a rhinestone in the center, and voilà, you're a nail artist! This textured effect is a very simple and effective way of jazzing up your nails. However, it can be quite tricky if you're not competent with both your hands, so going to a nail salon to have the professionals work their magic is always a good way to go.

Nail jewelry is also growing increasingly popular, from stuck-on jewels to nail piercings. If it's jewels you want, there are plenty of ready-made, detailed designs available on the market, and all you need to do is simply peel them off and stick them on. The vibrant colors and eye-catching embellishments of Indian-inspired designs (think *Slumdog Millionaire*

actress Freida Pinto's John Galliano dress at the Academy Awards) have been very popular.

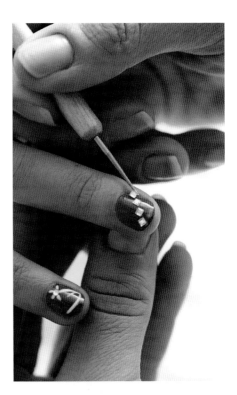

## Pro Tip

Longer nails carry more intricate designs better, as there is more space on the nail to add the design to.

# BASIC TOOLS

Here is a list of some of the tools and equipment you will need to put together a nail art kit and get going with some creative designs. In addition to nail polishes and paints, there is a huge selection of rhinestones, gems, glitter dusts, transfers, and paints to choose from. You're only limited by your own imagination and, of course, your own creativity and ability. Here is a list of items you could start out with, but keep your eyes open; in this rapidly evolving area of the market, new products, concepts, and ideas are being launched all the time.

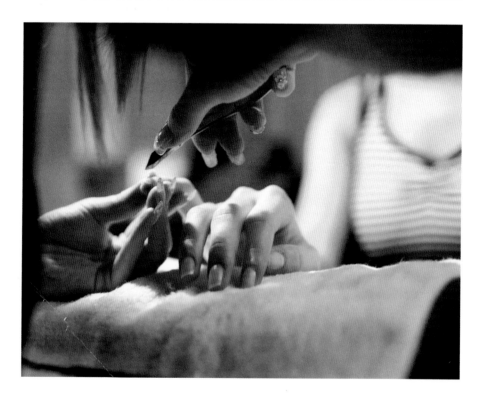

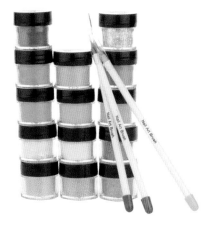

# Nail paints

Unlike nail polish, nail paint is usually acrylic, and these nontoxic, water-based acrylic paints are denser in color than nail polishes. A selection of primary colors, opalescent, pearlescent neon, and metallic colors would be ideal. Acrylics are easy to work with and a deep vibrant color is achievable.

## Nail art brushes

A selection will be needed, so try a liner brush for precision detailing, a long striping brush for creating straight lines, and a fan brush for creating any brushed or sweeping effects across the nail. Other brushes that might be useful include a glitter dust brush and a shading brush for texturing and blending colors together.

## Marbling and dotting tools

Available in a variety of sizes, the most popular is a double-ended tool, which has two metallic balls on either end of the handle; one ball is small and the other slightly larger. It is useful for creating dots, marbled designs, and swirls; detailing flowers and petals; and blending colors.

# Color-shapers

Available in a wide variety of shapes, sizes, and hardnesses. The pointed shaper is useful for creating dots and swirls; the cup shaper creates teardrops and half-circles; and the angled chisel shaper can define straight lines or half-circles.

## Transfers

These come in a variety of options, including water-release transfers and self-adhesive transfers, and can transform a nail in seconds. Designs can be very intricate and more detailed than anything you could do by hand.

## Tweezers

A must for picking up and securing striping tape, transfers, and tiny gems.

## Scissors

A must-have item. Useful for cutting lace, fiberglass, silk, and other fine materials.

## Sponges

Useful for creating texture and stippled effects.

## Foils

These can create some really pretty designs and the metallic finish is available in a variety of colors, textures, and patterns. Attach with foil adhesive, place with the pattern facing upward, and then rub onto the nail with a thumb or cotton swab. For best results, wait for the adhesive to become transparent.

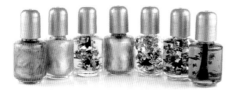

## Polish-secure items

To liven up any design, use two coats of polish and top coat and embed your rhinestones, flat-stones, pearls, or glitter dust. The polish will come up the sides, gripping the item, securing it, and ensuring a long-lasting effect. If you want to add a quick-drying top coat, just remember it might dull your gems.

### Rhinestones
Available in a variety of shapes, sizes, and colors, these polish-secure items adhere to wet polish. The use of one stone to complete a design can be very effective.

### Flat-stones
These are flatter versions of the rhinestones that won't knock off, and are smaller and less expensive. They are also polish-secure, but be aware that some cheaper makes lose their color when you apply your top coat, so test beforehand.

### Glitter dust
A fine, sparkly powder that can be very effective when applied to a nail design. Apply with a sable brush.

## Striping tape

This comes in all sorts of colors, including metallic finishes. Nonadhesive striping tape needs to be gently pressed into wet nail polish and may need a little adhesive to secure the ends once they have been cut. Some are self-adhesive, so they will need to be cut and pressed onto dry polish and have a top coat applied to keep the tape in place.

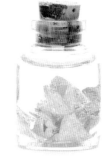

## Gold and silver leaf

Delicate and very fragile to work with, leaf will adhere to wet polish and is probably best applied in small pieces. Trying to create a smooth effect with the foils is impossible—creases are inevitable.

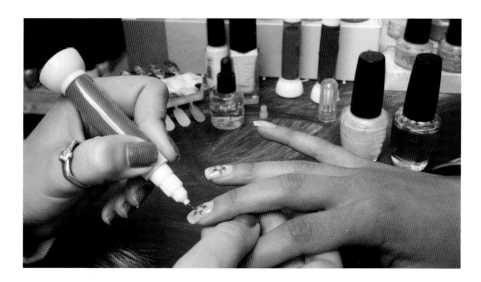

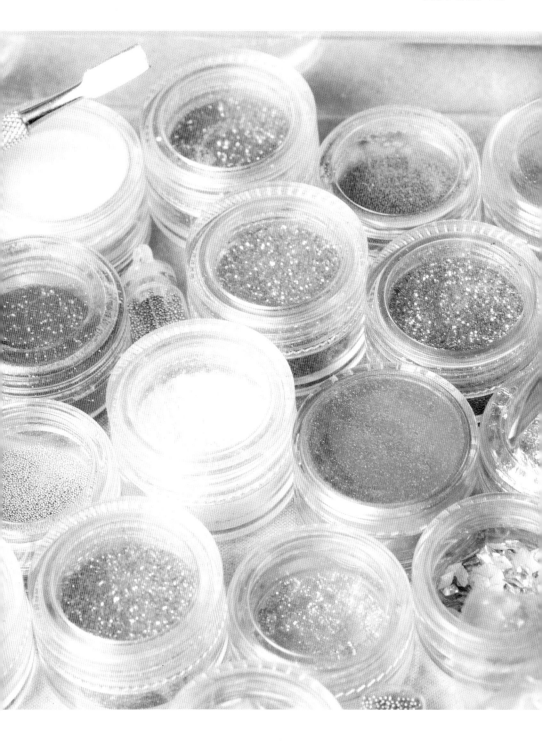

# FREEHAND DESIGN

Freehand design is probably the easiest place to start because you are not reliant on expensive equipment and the products and techniques are easily achieved. Experimentation is essential. These ideas are simply guidelines to get you started—so build up your repertoire and get going.

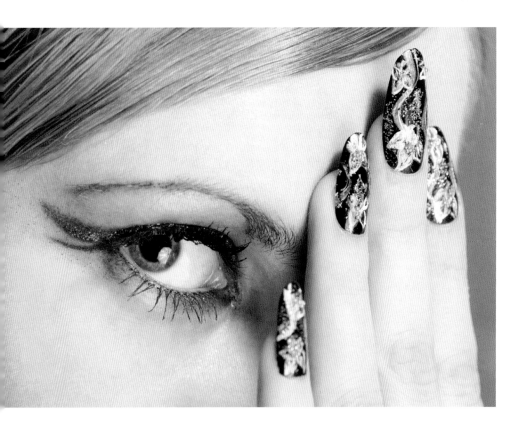

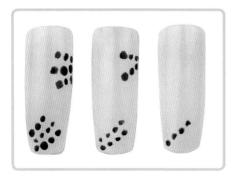

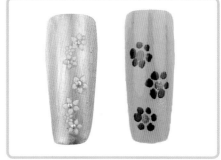

# Abstract dots

Simple and quick to achieve, all you need is a steady hand, a simple design idea, and a marbling tool, or something similar, to pick up and place the paint dots. Using a brush will result in an uneven finish.

## Equipment

Base coat, preferred nail polish color, contrasting color paint or nail polish, marbling tool, or pointed color-shaper, and top coat.

1 Apply base coat to all ten nails.
2 Apply two coats of preferred nail polish, ensuring good coverage of each nail.
3 Place the large end of the marbling tool into the chosen contrasting acrylic paint and dot your chosen pattern onto the nail, starting at the lower left-hand corner.
4 Use either the same size dots or varying sizes to make up your design. If you want the dots to gradually decrease in size, you should dot once into the paint and then dot three or more dots onto the nail before reapplying paint.
5 Allow paint to dry thoroughly before applying a top coat for protection.

# Daisy flowers

Flowers are really simple to do and look very effective, with minimal effort required. By dragging a brush through each dot, you can extend the petals. For a glam look, you can enhance the daisies with diamonds or pearls—highly effective on a French manicure. Try combining with linear stalks in a contrasting color for a floral bouquet.

## Equipment

Base coat, preferred nail polish color, contrasting color nail paint or polish, marbling tool or pointed color-shaper, and top coat.

1 Apply base coat to all ten nails.
2 Apply two coats of preferred polish, ensuring good coverage on all nails.
3 Load the large end of a marbling tool or pointed color-shaper with chosen shade of paint or nail polish and place five dots to create a flower shape. Reload the tool between each dot so that the dots are the same size. Repeat the dots diagonally across the nail.
4 Using a contrasting color of paint, dot into the middle of each daisy to create the center. You could also use a rhinestone or flat-stone here instead of paint.
5 Allow paint to dry thoroughly. Apply two coats of top coat for protection.

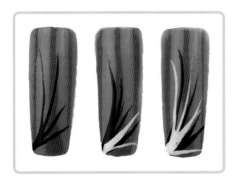

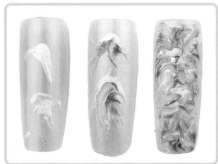

# Two-color stripe from corner

Graphic and simple to achieve, all this look requires is a steady hand.

## Equipment

Base coat, chosen nail polish color, striping brush, white and black nail paint, and top coat.

**1** Apply base coat to all ten nails.
**2** Apply two coats of preferred polish, ensuring even coverage on all nails.
**3** Load your striping brush with black paint. Place the brush in the bottom left corner, and pull it vertically across the nail in one sweeping movement. Reload the brush and make two smaller lines on either side of the first. Don't try to paint this with the tip of the brush because the result will be shaky and uneven. Instead, turn the brush horizontally and pull the brush through and up for a straight, bold, steady line.
**4** With white paint loaded onto a clean brush, repeat the movements, placing the white stripes between the black stripes for a graphic contrasted effect.
**5** Allow the paint to dry thoroughly before applying a layer of top coat to seal and protect.

# Marbling

With contrasting colors for maximum impact, you can use acrylic colors to allow you more time to create your design. There is no reason why you can't work with nail enamel, although you will have less time to perfect your design because it dries so quickly.

## Equipment

Base coat, chosen nail polish color, two or three contrasting color nail paints or polishes, marbling tool, and top coat.

**1** Apply base coat to all ten nails.
**2** Apply two coats of preferred polish, ensuring good coverage on all nails.
**3** Using the large end of the marbling tool, place drops of contrasting nail paints onto the corner of the nail.
**4** Clean marbling tool.
**5** Using both ends of the tool, swirl one color of paint into the other to create the marbling effect. Each end of the tool will give you a different-sized swirl.
**6** Allow paint to dry completely before applying two coats of top coat for protection.

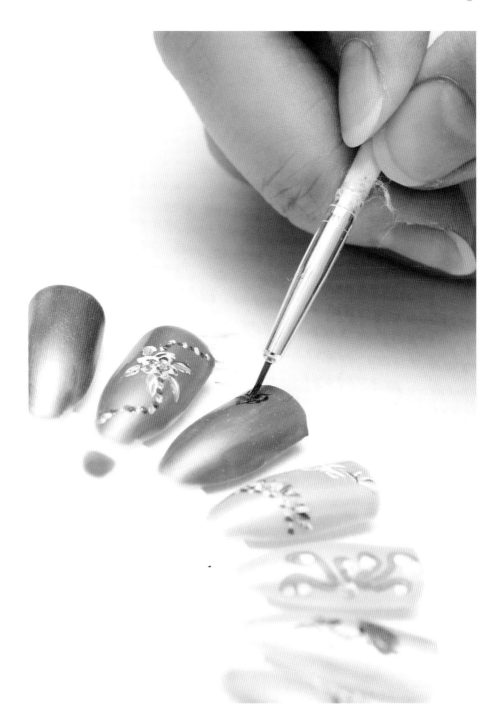

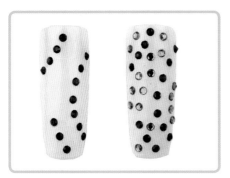

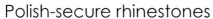

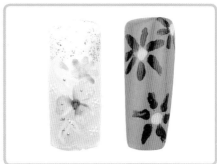

# Polish-secure rhinestones

With endless possibilities, this bling look is fun, quick, and easy to achieve. Just make sure the wet polish secures the rhinestones.

## Equipment
Base coat, preferred nail polish shade, two colors of rhinestones, orangewood stick tipped with a reusable pressure-sensitive adhesive putty or tweezers, and top coat.

**1** Apply base coat to all ten nails.
**2** Apply two coats of preferred polish, ensuring good coverage on all nails.
**3** Allow to dry thoroughly before applying two coats of top coat for protection.
**4** Use the tipped orangewood stick or tweezers to place the rhinestones and create an abstract pattern. Press each rhinestone gently into the top coat, making sure the sides are immersed in the wet nail polish to ensure adequate adhesion.
**5** Change to the other color of rhinestones to complete the pattern.
**6** You might need to apply small dots of top coat to secure the stones in place as you are working. Allow to dry thoroughly.
**7** Apply a top coat, but remember that some top coats will dull the glint of the rhinestones.

# Larger freehand flowers

Pretty and feminine flowers are easy to do. By using a flatter brush and a rotation motion, you can create rounder petals, while a longer bristled brush pulled through the stroke will create pointed petals.

## Equipment
Base coat, preferred nail polish shade, contrasting colors of nail paint or polish, and top coat. You could also add glitter dust to finish off.

**1** Apply base coat to all ten nails.
**2** Apply two coats of preferred polish, ensuring good coverage on all nails.
**3** Create the flower centers (dots) with the marbling tool and contrasting nail colors (or you can add a gemstone center if you wish).
**4** Using brush loaded with chosen contrast shade, place the brush for each petal and then pull outward to create a pointed shape. Or rotate to create the circular effect of rounded petals, pulling the brush outward so most of the paint remains in the center of the flower.
**5** Repeat until you have your desired pattern. You can also achieve interesting results by combining two colors for each petal—place one half of the brush in one color and the other half into another color. Keep the brush in an upright position on the nail, and turn clockwise to mix the paint together—the resulting blend creates a perfect two-toned petal. All it takes is a little practice.
**6** Finish off with leaves and shading if desired.
**7** Apply one coat of top coat to seal and protect.

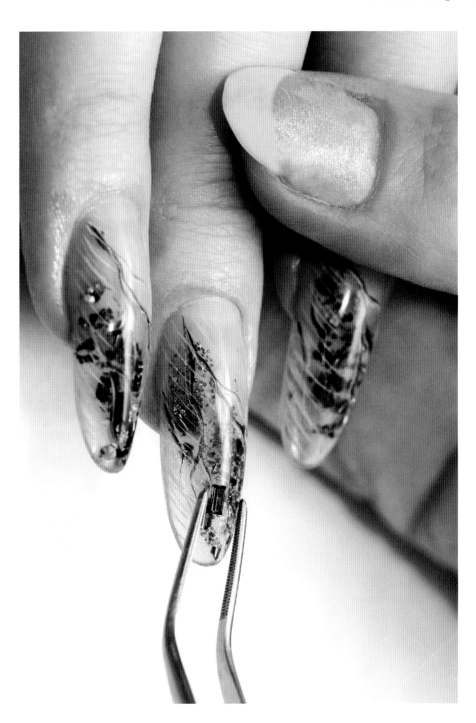

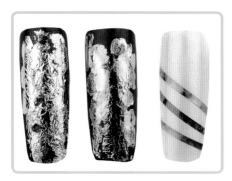
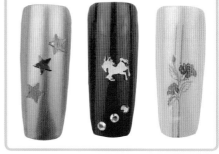

## Foiling

Another easy technique using foiled tape. Some foils have designs on them and just need to be applied to a painted nail. Foil can be purchased in rolls or sheets.

### Equipment
Base coat, nail polish color of choice, foils, foil adhesive, cotton swabs, scissors, and top coat.

**1** Apply base coat to all ten nails. You can leave the nail clear, but a base coat is preferable as the moisture and oils from the natural nail will reduce the bond of the foils and adhesive.
**2** Apply two coats of preferred polish, ensuring even coverage on all nails.
**3** Once the enamel has dried, apply foil adhesive sparingly where you want the foil to be applied. The adhesive is initially white but becomes clear after a while.
**4** When the adhesive has become transparent, press the foil (with pattern up) onto the nail. Rub with a cotton swab to ensure adhesion and remove quickly. The decorated foil strips will adhere wherever the glue was applied, making for quick and easy nail art. You can also create patterns with the adhesive because the foil sticks only where the adhesive has been applied. The backing is pulled off, leaving the foil behind.
**5** The foil needs a special sealer, as most top coats will destroy the delicate layer. Several layers of sealer should be applied to keep it intact.

## Transfers and tapes

Many lovely tapes and transfers are available to apply to nails. This ready-made nail art is quick and easy to apply and can be very effective. Some transfers and decals need to be soaked off with water; simply apply a few drops to the back of the transfer to soak through. When saturated, the transfer will slide off the backing and stick straight to the nail. Tapes are available in all sorts of colors and patterns. Usually adhesive-backed, they are easy to apply and simply need to be cut to size.

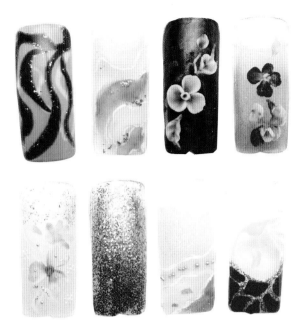

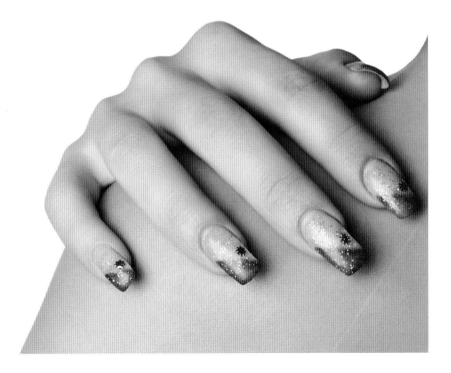

# AIRBRUSH METHOD

With more and more salons investing in the necessary equipment, airbrushing is becoming increasingly popular. The airbrush itself has numerous applications, including tanning solutions, temporary tattoos, and makeup application. Nail art is just another arena where airbrush application offers an accurate, detailed application that takes half the time of traditional hand-painting. In fact, airbrushing is rapidly overtaking traditional nail polishing in many salons. With the right equipment it is perfectly possible for anyone to learn how to use the airbrush method—all it takes is a steady hand and a lot of practice.

Airbrushing is a method of applying or spraying a fine mist of color on the nails in layers using compressed air. Initially used by graphic artists, usage has now extended to the cosmetic world where airguns are very popular for fake tan application and nail art. Unlike basic nail art, however, airbrushing requires costly equipment. It might look easy but it requires great skill. Once mastered, it will help speed up your design application, opening up endless creative options. Perseverance is crucial, and ultimately, you'll be able to work on natural nails, nail enhancements, and even toenails.

The airbrush itself is a small, air-operated tool that sprays acrylic nail paints by a process of nebulization. It looks very easy in the hands of an expert, but you'll need to experiment before investing. Remember that proficiency takes time and many hours of practice. A practical training course is highly recommended if you want to become adept. There are two types of airbrushes available: the single action and the more traditional double or dual action. In a dual action brush, the trigger or lever has a dual purpose: the first action allows the air to flow and the second action engages the paint supply and enables it to flow freely—the further the trigger is pressed, the more is released. More difficult to control, this type of airbrush ultimately allows for greater versatility, control, and creativity.

You will need an electrical compressor. An air pressure regulator is also important, as it allows you to select the required air pressure, determined by the applications you will be using it for. For instance: makeup 7 PSI (pounds per square inch); body art 15 PSI; tanning 20 PSI; and nail art 35 PSI. You will also need the right paint. There are two types of paint available for nail art: a water-based paint that contains acrylic color and dissolves in water (usually opaque, although pearlescent and metallic formulas are also available); and acrylic-based paint which, has a higher concentration of acrylic paint and is denser and brighter in coloration, but not as easy to remove from skin and clothing if you make a mess. The airbrush has delicate parts that need to be kept clean and lubricated. Correct cleaning is crucial. Always use the recommended cleanser appropriate for the paints you are using and clean thoroughly after each use—any paint left in the paint container will dry out and flake off, leaving the nozzle blocked and inoperable.

Airbrushing is all about layering color—laying one color over another, resulting in different colors. Wonderful effects can be achieved by merging two colors and effects like color-fades or gradient blends where the colors merge, creating dimension and depth. There are times where you will need to maintain the true color of your paint; this is when you spray onto a white base.

Airbrushed nail color will last longer than traditional nail enamel, since it is a thinner coating. Any airbrush paint that is not sealed to the nail may be washed away later. Secure one or two coats of protective airbrush sealer, then cleanse the fingers or toes as per the manufacturer's instructions. Use an orangewood stick wrapped in a cotton pad and saturated with nail polish remover to remove any paint sealed to the skin.

# Advantages

Detailed designs are possible in a fraction of the time hand-painting would require; acrylic paints are more affordable; lines are more accurate; and you are more likely to achieve a smooth, professional finish. Airbrushing dries instantly, so intricate designs can be achieved much more quickly.

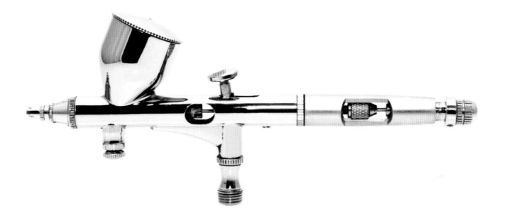

# Stencils and masks

From the simplicity of a French manicure to the most complex designs, stencils can assist in building up the layers. Used either in part or as a whole image, they help speed up the process. Stencils, pre-cut shapes in thin plastic, are usually pliable plastic and are used either in part by just using the edge or the whole when an entire pattern is cut out. By varying the distance the stencil is held from the nail, you can create sharp or soft edges. Overlapping, rotating, and repeating shapes will mean that the possibilities are endless. You can make your own stencils with masking tape or sticky-backed acetate; draw your design onto the masking material and cut it out with a sharp craft knife. Consider the following: lace or net overlays create a beautiful textured effect; your thumb could act as a stencil when spraying a basic French manicure; you could use the straight edge of a business card to create a chevron French (a French manicure with the tips painted in a V-shape); or you could even use leaves as masks—the list is endless.

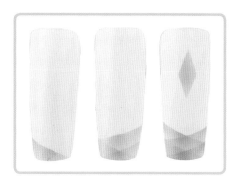

# French manicure alternative

## Equipment

Airbrush, compressor, cleaner and cleaning station, base coat, a light shade and a slightly darker acrylic color of your choice, airbrush sealant, stencil or mask with straight edge, cut-out diamond-shape stencil, top coat.

1 Apply base coat to all ten nails.
2 Spray lightest shade on the entire nail, ensuring even coverage.
3 Once dry, apply the straight edge of the stencil diagonally over the free edge at the corner of the nail and spray with a darker shade. Make sure it has dried before moving the stencil.
4 Move the stencil to the opposite corner of the free edge and repeat.
5 Move the stencil up the nail and repeat the process on both sides.
6 Position and spray the cut-out diamond shape in the middle of the nail plate.
7 Seal with airbrush sealant and apply top coat for extra protection and shine.

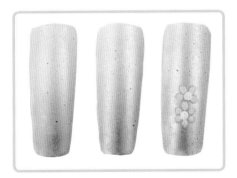

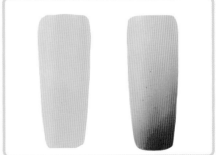

# Color fade with flower

## Equipment

Airbrush, compressor, cleaner and cleaning station, base coat, chosen base color, metallic color of choice, airbrush sealant, and top coat.

**1** Apply base coat to all ten nails.
**2** Spray the lightest color over the entire nail, ensuring even coverage.
**3** Create the color fade by spraying on the darker color, starting from the right free edge and back again, this time closer to the free edge.
By setting a less fine spray, you can control the size of the droplets.
**4** Using your marbling tool (see page 159), pick up the selected color and place a dot at the center of flower. Change color and place another dot, replenishing paint on the tool after each dot. Place five petals around the central dot and repeat for the second flower.
**5** Seal the design with airbrush sealant.
**6** Apply top coat for protection and shine.

# Two-color fades

## Equipment

Airbrush, compressor, cleaner and cleaning station, base coat, chosen base color, two contrasting acrylic colors of choice, airbrush with sealant, and top coat.

**1** Apply base coat to all ten nails.
**2** Spray the lightest color over the entire nail, ensuring even coverage.
**3** Create the color fade by spraying the darker color, starting from the right free edge and back again, this time closer to the free edge, ensuring a denser coverage on the outer edge. This can serve as a perfect base for a number of effective designs.
**4** Seal the design with airbrush sealant.
**5** Apply top coat for protection and shine.

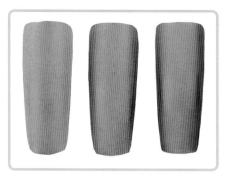

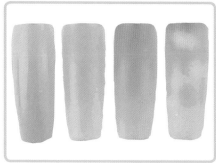

## Contouring color

### Equipment
Base coat, two contrasting acrylic paints in preferred color shades, airbrush sealant, and top coat.

**1** Apply base coat to all ten nails.
**2** Spray the lightest color over the entire nail, ensuring even coverage.
**3** Spray the darker color down the sides of each nail, taking care that both sides are even in width and match all ten fingers. This is a great way of elongating and refining the contours, and can be a very effective base for all sorts of creative designs.
**4** Seal with airbrush sealant.
**5** Apply top coat for protection and shine.

## Color fade with clouds

### Equipment
Base coat, pale blue, mid-blue, dark blue, and white airbrush paints, airbrush sealant, piece of torn tissue used as mask, and top coat.

**1** Apply base coat to all ten nails.
**2** Spray lightest shade on all nails, ensuring even coverage.
**3** Start spraying on the right-hand side of the cuticle with the mid-blue paint. Work from side to side diagonally across the nail, halfway down the nail and back up to the free edge. Repeat, but this time work only a quarter of the way down and back to the free edge. Repeat on all nails.
**4** Spray the dark blue just at the top corner, hardly touching the nail.
**5** Spray small bursts of white randomly to create the clouds. For added definition, you could spray onto a torn strip of tissue as a mask, moving the tissue down to create denser clouds by layering.
**6** Seal the design with sealant.
**7** Apply top coat for protection and shine.

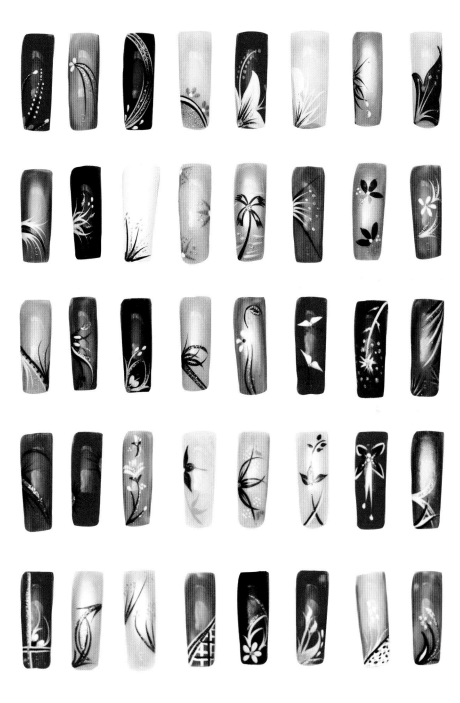

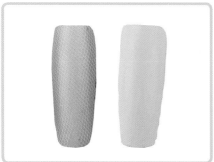

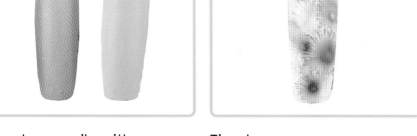

# Contour nails with masked netting

This pretty effect streamlines and lengthens wide nails, and the netting creates a subtle visual effect that adds another dimension.

## Equipment
Base coat, three contrasting colored paints, netting for masked effect, airbrush sealant, and top coat.

**1** Apply base coat to all ten nails.
**2** Spray the pale green, or the palest of your preferred color choices, onto all nails, ensuring even coverage.
**3** Airbrush the darker shade down both sides of the nail, ensuring that both sides are evenly matched on all ten fingers. Be sure to create a shade effect along the contour to create the illusion of slimmer and longer nails.
**4** Airbrush the netting to create a three-dimensional effect, repeating on all fingers.
**5** Seal with airbrush sealant.
**6** Apply top coat for strength, protection, and shine.

# Tie dye

This pretty splotched effect is simple to do and takes no time at all. In soft pastel colors, it's the ideal spring or summer accessory.

## Equipment
Base coat, three shades of airbrush paints, airbrush sealant, and top coat.

**1** Apply base coat to all ten nails.
**2** Airbrush the palest color over the entire nail plate, ensuring even coverage.
**3** Hold the airbrush at a 90° angle, loaded with the second color, and spray directly onto the nail. Press the trigger down and lift the airbrush straight up releasing the trigger at the same time. This will create a splotched effect.
**4** Repeat the first color randomly over the nail and then on the remaining nails.
**5** Change colors and layer the splotches over the entire nail, making sure each layer is dry before spraying the next to avoid losing definition.
**6** Seal with airbrush sealant before applying a top coat for protection and shine.

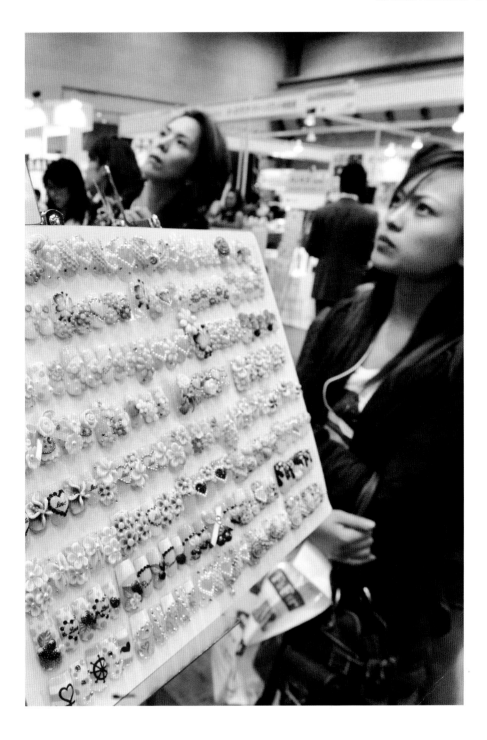

# COLORED ACRYLICS

Nail acrylic art has caught the imagination of the fashion world because of its versatility and dynamism. With the wide variety of colored acrylic powders available, you can create just about any color you want. This method can be used if you want a more permanent solution, rather than using polish colors that have to be reapplied each time. Colored acrylic is ideal for the purpose of creating three-dimensional effects for nails, and all sorts of items can be embedded, such as leaves, small stars and hearts, tiny pearls, crushed shells, dried flowers, and beads to really enhance your designs.

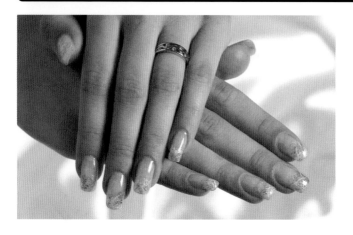

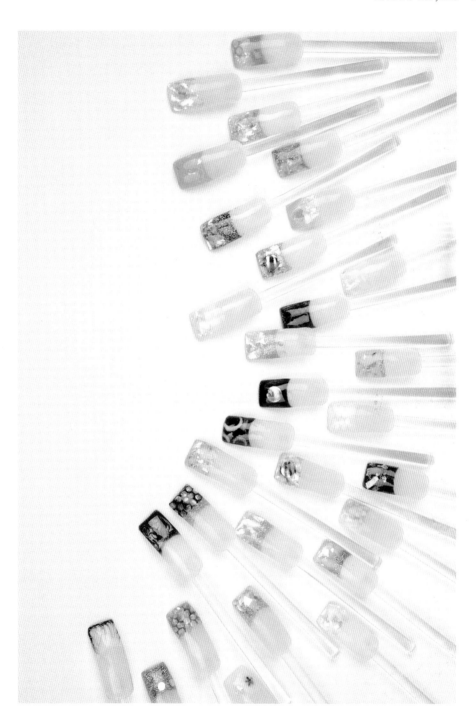

# Acrylic reverse method

This method is becoming increasingly popular, as it is quick and efficient. Although it can seem a little heavy, all excess acrylic is filed off in the final stages. It also offers a long-lasting method of embedding jewels, glitter, crushed shell, and the like.

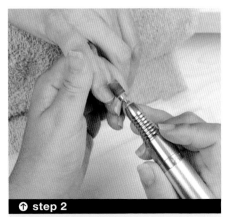

**⬆ step 2**

Buff the natural nail surfaces and file free edges to shape.

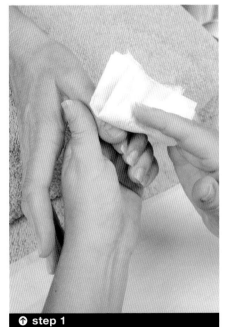

**⬆ step 1**

Prepare the nail by carefully removing all traces of cuticle from the nail plate and then dehydrating.

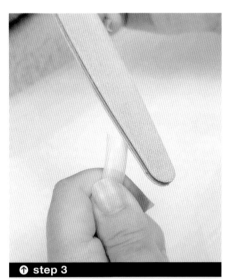

**⬆ step 3**

Shape the tips with a nail file and smooth rough edges away.

### ● step 4

Apply a drop of nail adhesive to the nail tip, which is held at a 45° angle. Place the top of the tip at the free edge, roll back, then press down and hold in place.

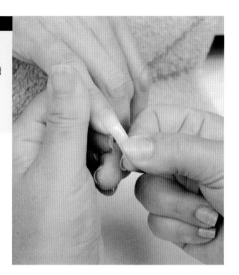

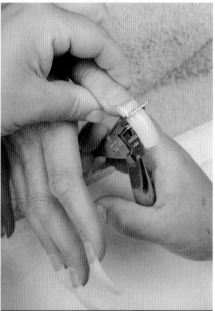

### ⬆ step 5

Trim the tips with a special nail trimmer. Blend the tip seam where it joins the nail and shape the free edge with a medium to fine file.

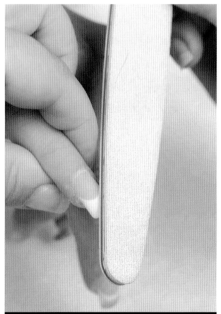

### ⬆ step 6

Buff the nails and smooth carefully. Dust off any nail particles with a manicure brush and scrub nails clean with acetone to remove any oil and contaminants.

### ➔ step 7

Apply one coat of acrylic bonding agent or primer to the natural nail to help bond the keratin with the polymer.

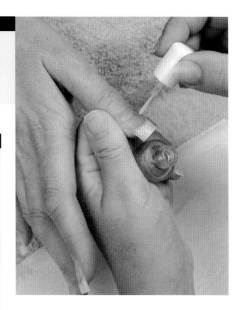

### step 8

Pour acrylic liquid (monomer) and acrylic powder (polymer) into separate glass containers. Dip the brush into the liquid, submerging the bristles of your brush into the liquid to free it from air pockets and then press against the dish to release any excess. Wipe the brush carefully on a paper towel. (Most acrylics are now self-leveling and the consistency that works best is when the acrylic pearl is a matte finish.)

### step 9

Dip the tip of the brush gently into the pink powder, until it has gathered as much powder as the brush can hold, and the pearl is large enough to shape the entire nail plate from cuticle to smile line, excluding the tip.

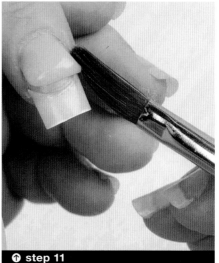

### step 10

Apply the large pink pearl at the center of what is left of the exposed natural nail and press the bead in the center, nudging it back to the cuticle, then drawing the brush back over the product. This will ensure that there is no ridge at the cuticle, which must lie flush with the nail plate, and will save unnecessary filing in this delicate area. Press the bead to either side and smooth over to give even coverage.

### ➊ step 11

Hold sidewall evenly and press acrylic across the free edge and up to the opposite side of the smile.

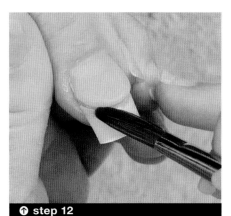

**↑ step 12**

By holding the tip of the brush at a 45° angle behind the smile line, you will carve a groove at the smile to ensure proper groove depth. This will prevent the white from shadowing through the pink powder.

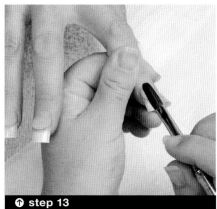

**↑ step 13**

While this method looks heavy, most of the acrylic is worked away with an electric file. Ensure the product has been laid evenly across the nail plate; if the pearl is too large, it can make the upper arch too high and result in excessive filing. Pat the arch down to level the existing product at the apex.

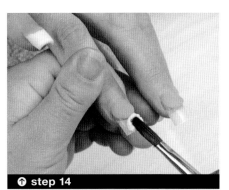

**↑ step 14**

The second pearl, using the white to create a French tip effect, should be laid behind the smile line to fill in any unevenness. Make sure the pearl is not too big, as this can make the upper arch too high. Use the flat surface of the brush to contour the acrylic nail to match the shape of the natural nail when laying down your cuticle area. Repeat on each finger.

**➔ step 15**

Using a 180-grit file shape the free edge into the preferred shape. When shaping the free edge, you can create square, oval, or square-oval by holding the file at specific angles.

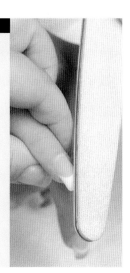

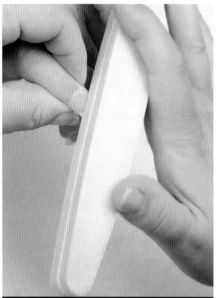

**⬆ step 16**

Use your 180-grit sponge file and buff the entire surface. Then use a 240-grit white file and file the entire area, concentrating on the cuticle edge.

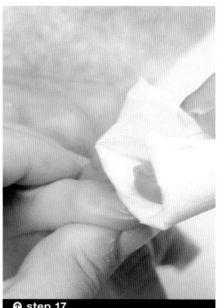

**⬆ step 17**

Remove dust and wipe off.

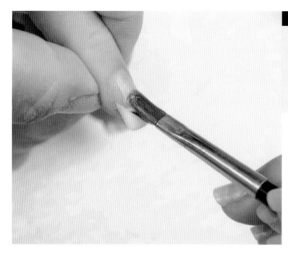

**⬅ step 18**

Apply a thin coat of gel and place under the light to cure completely before applying cuticle oil.

# French striped dot

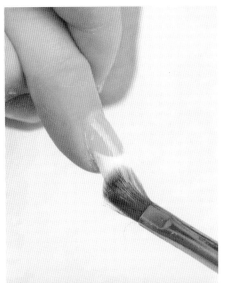

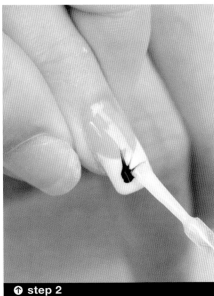

### ⬆ step 1

Continuing with the method from step 17, apply a thin coat of gel and, before placing under the light for curing, continue applying your design.

### ⬆ step 2

Place a dot of black acrylic paint on the outer right corner, then place your striping brush into the dot and pull it through, creating three separate stripes in the process. You could always add a flat gem for more drama.

### step 3

Place under the light to cure completely before applying cuticle oil.

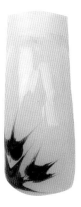

# Dramatic pull-through

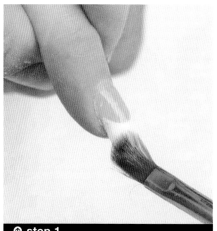

### ⬆ step 1

Continuing with the method from step 17 on page 184, apply a thin coat of gel and, before placing under the light for curing, continue applying your design.

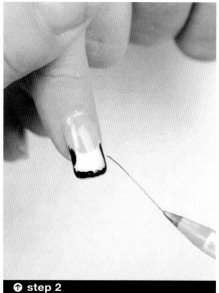

### ⬆ step 2

Apply black acrylic around the outer edges of the free edge.

### ➔ step 3

Pull your striping brush through the black paint a few times, creating a fringed effect.

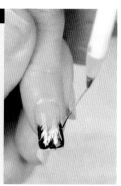

### step 4

Place under the light to cure completely before applying cuticle oil.

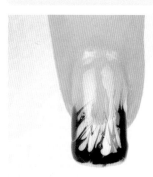

# Black net inlay

## step 1

The second pearl (using the white to create a French tip effect) should be laid behind the smile line to fill in any unevenness. Make sure the pearl is not too big, as this can make the upper arch too high. Ensure the flat surface of the brush contours to the shape of the natural nail when laying down your cuticle area. Repeat on each finger.

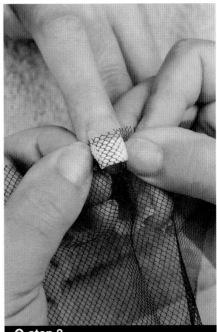

## ↑ step 2

While still wet, place a piece of netting into the white and press down, embedding it into the acrylic. Then lift and remove, leaving an indentation.

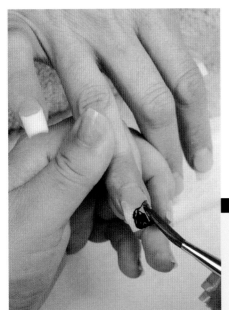

## ← step 3

Apply black-colored acrylic gel over the indentation, making sure you press it into the impression. Work from edge to edge and allow to dry.

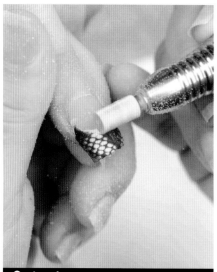

**⬆ step 4**

Use your 180-grit sponge file, or electric file, and buff the entire surface. Then use a 240-grit white file and file the entire area, concentrating on the cuticle edge. This will remove excess black acrylic, revealing the net pattern.

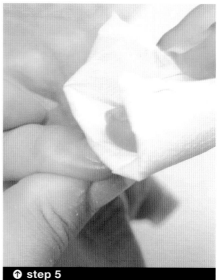

**⬆ step 5**

Remove dust and wipe off.

**➔ step 6**

Apply a thin coat of gel, sprinkle with glitter, and place under the light to cure completely before applying cuticle oil.

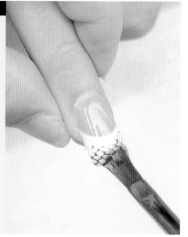

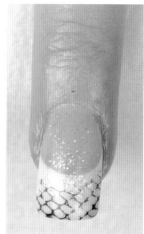

# Polka dots

This playful and funky look carries on from the basic reverse method application (page 180) and picks up from step 13.

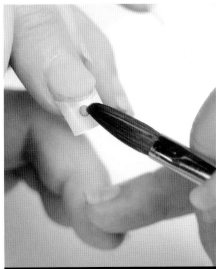

**⬆ step 1**

Create a tiny ball of acrylic using bright pink powder. Place onto free edge in the center, patting it into place to flatten slightly.

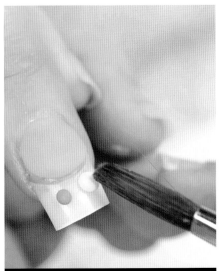

**⬆ step 2**

Create a slightly larger ball of acrylic using bright yellow powder and place it on the free edge to the right of the pink dot, patting into place to flatten slightly.

### ● step 3

Create an even larger ball of acrylic using bright green powder and place it to the left of the pink dot, patting into place and flattening slightly.

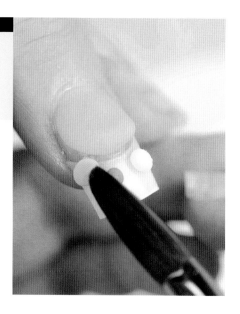

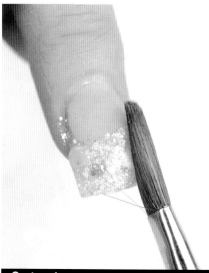

### ① step 4

Fill with clear acrylic gel dipped into glitter along the free edge, working into the smile line and gently drawing the gel across the entire area.

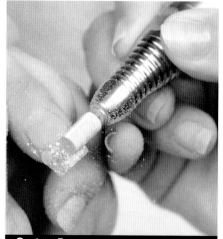

### ① step 5

Using your 180-grit sponge file, or electric file, file and buff the entire surface. Then use a 240-grit white file and file the entire area, concentrating on the free edge and maintaining the right shape.

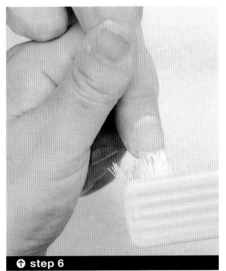

**⬆ step 6**

Remove dust and brush off.

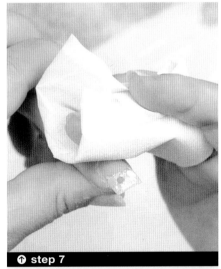

**⬆ step 7**

Wipe off any residue.

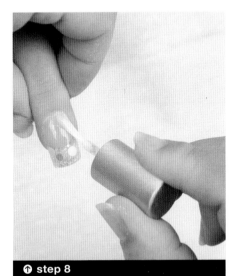

**⬆ step 8**

Apply a thin coat of gel and place under the light to cure completely before applying cuticle oil.

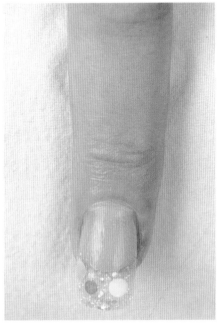

# Asymmetrical green glitter

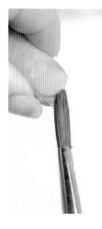

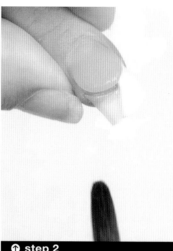

### ◉ step 1

The second pearl (half the size in this instance, using the white to create a French tip effect) should be laid behind the smile line to fill in any unevenness. Place it on the right side of the nail, working outward to the edge. Ensure the flat surface of the brush contours to the shape of the natural nail when laying down your sidewall.

### ◉ step 2

Place the edge of the brush on the left side of this pearl, straightening the line, thus creating an asymmetrical wedge.

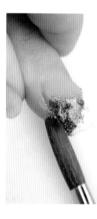

### ◉ step 3

Fill the other side with clear acrylic gel dipped into green glitter. Check and maintain the sidewalls, making sure you fill up to and include the smile line.

### ◉ step 4

Place a rhinestone gem into the green glitter gel, pressing it in firmly with your orange stick. Be sure to embed the gem in the gel, so when filing you won't scratch or remove the gem.

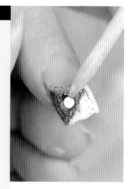

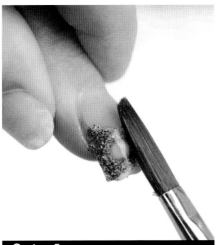

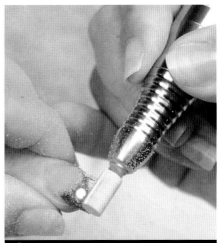

**⬆ step 5**

Cover and smooth over with clear gel, sculpting and shaping the nail as you work.

**⬆ step 6**

Using a 180-grit sponge file, or electric file, shape the free edge, then file and buff the entire surface. Then use a 240-grit white file and file the entire area, concentrating on the cuticle edge.

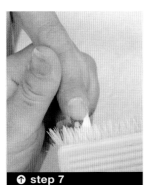

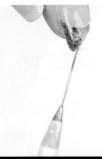

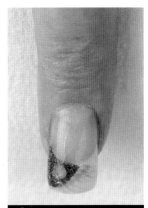

**⬆ step 7**

Remove dust and wipe off.

**⬆ step 8**

Apply a thin line of yellow acrylic paint along a diagonal line and allow to dry. Then change to green and paint a line, pulling the brush through this wet line to create a fringed effect.

**⬆ step 9**

Apply a thin coat of gel and place under the light to cure completely before applying cuticle oil.

# Double-smile gray and pink glitter

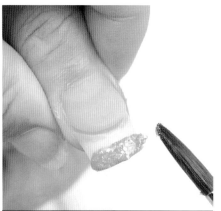

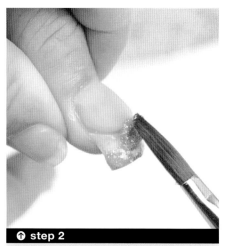

### ⊙ step 2

For the third ball, use a silvery gray glitter gel and lay it behind the smile line to fill in and cover the pink strip. Make sure the pearl is not too big, as this can make the upper arch too high. Ensure the flat surface of the brush contours to the shape of the natural nail when laying down your cuticle area. Repeat on each finger.

### ⊙ step 1

In this case, create the second pearl with bright pink glitter gel, placed onto the free edge. Paint it on following the smile line but cover only half of the tip.

### ➜ step 3

Apply a little transparent gel to combine and merge with the rest of the nail.

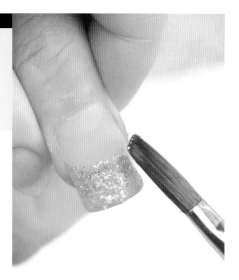

## step 4

Apply clear acrylic gel dipped into glitter along the free edge, working into the smile line, and gently drawing the gel across the entire area.

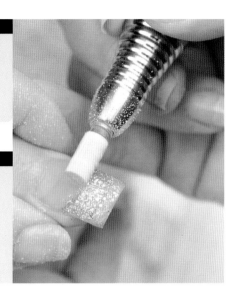

## ➔ step 5

Using your 180-grit sponge file, or electric file, buff and file the entire surface. Then use a 240-grit white file and file the entire area, concentrating on the free edge and maintaining the right shape.

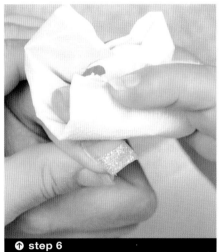

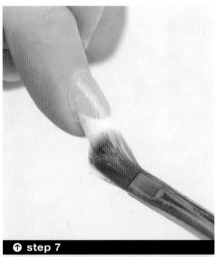

## ⬆ step 6

Remove dust and wipe off.

## ⬆ step 7

Apply a thin coat of gel.

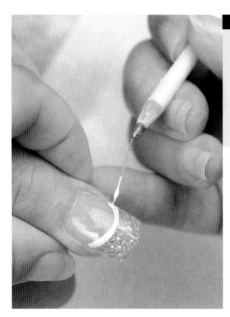

### ⟵ step 8

Apply a white line to the wet gel with your striping brush along the smile line.

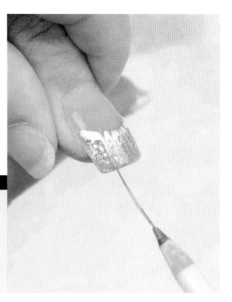

### ⟶ step 9

Drag the striping brush through the white line a few times, creating a fringed effect.

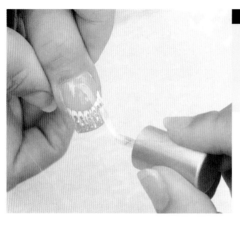

### ⟵ step 10

Place under the light to cure completely before applying cuticle oil.

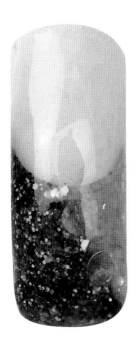
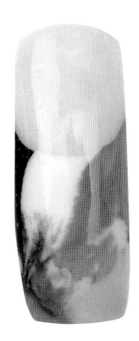
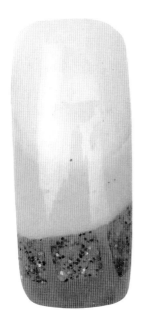
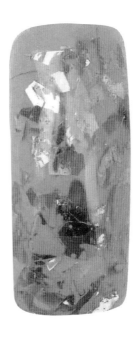

# Chapter **6**

# NAIL REMEDIES

Your nails are there to protect the delicate nerve endings of your toes and fingers. Knocks and trauma will cause damage to the nail bed. Deficiencies in certain vitamins and minerals, and fine chemical and hormone imbalances in the body also cause damage to the natural nail.

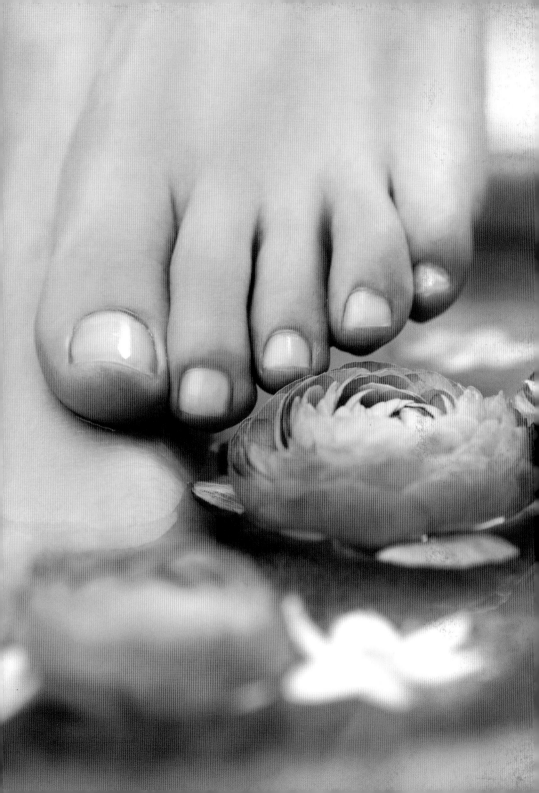

# NAIL SOLUTIONS

Look after your body and your nails stand a much better chance of growing to be strong, healthy, and straight. Looking at any visible changes on the nail surface will help you to assess chemical changes in the body. The following pages explain how you can treat these problems at home; but if in any doubt, consult your doctor.

Like good skin and thick hair, strong nails are a hereditary trait, although vitamin A and nail-strengthening supplements can help firm thin nails. Regular grooming, as well as brushing on a nail-strengthening formula, can also help prevent breakage. Clippers can bend and break the nails, so use scissors for trimming.

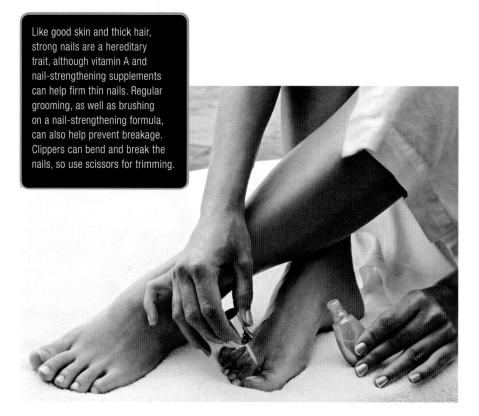

| Problem | Symptoms | Solution |
|---------|----------|----------|
| **Brittle nails** | Characterized by a vertical splitting or separation of the nail plate layers at the tip of the nail plate. In most cases, nail splitting is part of the natural aging process. This nail problem can also be the result of overexposure to water and chemical solvents such as household cleaning solutions. | Wear gloves whenever working with household cleaning solutions. |
| **Bruised nails** | These are those nails with spots of blood or bruises under the nail plate, caused by injury. New nail growth will depend on the extent of the damage. In some cases, the nail will fall off as part of the healing process. | Try increasing your zinc intake. Mild cases may be treated carefully by gently buffing to help smooth out furrows, or by filling with ridge-filler and covering with a polish of your choice. |
| **Contact dermatitis** | This is a reaction in the nail to contact with either irritants or allergens, such as monomers, adhesives, or primers. Symptoms include itching, redness, and dryness. Can be confused with psoriasis or onychomycosis. | Discontinue use of the irritating or allergenic material. Refer the problem to a dermatologist if it is unclear what is causing it. |
| **Hangnails** | These are small tears or splits in the nail plate or surrounding tissue. Usually the result of nail biting, they may also be caused by dry skin or injury. If untreated, they may tear and become raw, painful, and subject to infection. | Treat with an antiseptic if affected area is small. |

# FINGERNAIL DIAGNOSTICS

Our nails can change texture, color, thickness, and shape, and often these changes are reflective of our inner health. Monitor changes carefully and get the appropriate help.

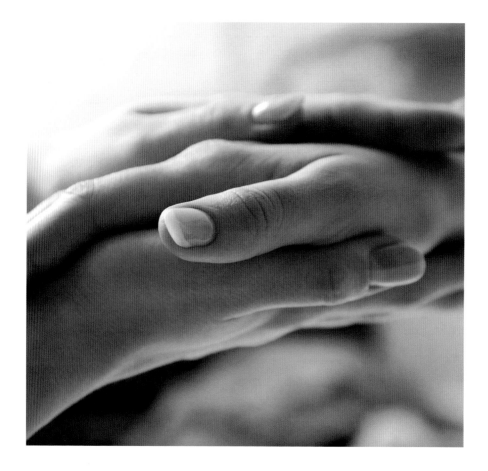

| Problem | Symptoms | Solution |
|---|---|---|
| **Vertical ridges** | These are also characteristic of aging, although not limited to the aged or elderly. As we age, the natural oil and moisture levels decline in the nail plate. | Ridged nails will improve through rehydration of the nail plate with twice daily applications of good-quality nail and cuticle oil containing jojoba and vitamin E. |
| **Furrows** | Furrows or corrugations are long ridges that run either lengthwise or across the nail. Lengthwise ridges can be caused by psoriasis and poor circulation. Ridges that run across the nail can be caused by conditions such as high fever, pregnancy, poor circulation, measles in childhood, a zinc deficiency in the body, or even frostbite. | Try increasing your zinc intake. Mild cases may be treated carefully by gently buffing to help smooth out furrows. Alternatively, fill with ridge filler and cover with a polish of your choice. |
| **Fungal or yeast infections** | A fungal or yeast infection can invade through a tear in the nail folds. It normally appears white or yellowish in color, and may also change the texture and shape of the nail. The fungus digests the keratin protein of which the nail plate is comprised. As the infection progresses, organic debris accumulates under the nail plate, often discoloring it. | Diagnosis is essential—once you have been diagnosed, ensure all the tools in your kit are sterilized. Stop wearing nail polish and artificial nails—they merely exacerbate the problem, as they contain chemicals that can damage the tissues of weak nails. Wear rubber gloves for household chores; any prolonged exposure to chemicals or even water will weaken the nails and cause damage. If the fungal infection persists, see a dermatologist; it might be a symptom of a medical condition like diabetes or low immune resistance. |
| **Leukonychia** | This consists of white spots on the nail plate. Leukonychia is often caused by a minor trauma to the nail bed or matrix, or it may be caused by tiny bubbles of air that are trapped in the nail plate layers because of trauma. Spots will grow out as the nail grows and will not affect a manicure or pedicure. | No need for treatment. |

# NAIL INFECTIONS AND DISEASES

These can be caused by a number of different conditions; if you have a badly infected nail, it is best to consult a dermatologist.

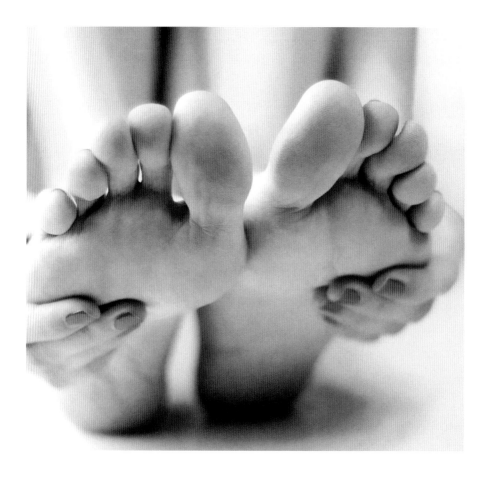

| Problem | Symptoms | Solution |
|---|---|---|
| **Contact dermatitis** | This is an allergic reaction to certain substances touching the skin. Symptoms are itching, redness, and dryness. When it affects nails and the surrounding skin, it is probably caused by irritants such as adhesives, monomers, or primers used to secure acrylic nails. Stop using the irritating substance or consult a dermatologist if you are unsure of the cause. | The condition may be confused with psoriasis or onychomycosis, which is an infectious disease caused by fungus, resulting in white patches that can be scraped off the nail, or yellowish streaks within the nail. |
| **Deformed nail plate** | A nail plate that is shaped like a spoon and is white and opaque is often caused by age, but can be also provide clues to common medical problem such as eczema, tumors, anemia, or chronic infection. The index, ring, and middle fingers are most affected. | Treat affected nails gently, as the nail plate will be fragile. See a doctor if you do suspect related medical problems. |
| **Hematoma** | Hematoma, or bruised nails, is a condition in which a clot of dried blood is formed between the nail plate and the nail bed. It varies in color from dark red to black, and in some cases the nail plate will separate and become infected. New growth will depend on the extent of the damage. It is usually caused by trauma from impact, such as being hit on the nail with a hammer, or friction from ill-fitting shoes (as is common with runners). | See your doctor. They might choose to relieve the pressure by puncturing the nail with a heated needle to prevent nail loss, but do not try doing this yourself as you could end up with an infection if you puncture the nail bed by mistake. |

| Problem | Symptoms | Solution |
|---------|----------|----------|
| **Melanonychia** | Usually associated with vertical pigmented brown or black stripes, or nail "moles" that form in the nail matrix. This sudden change on the nail plate could indicate a malignant melanoma or lesion that requires medical advice. That said, dark streaks are fairly frequent and a normal occurrence for dark-skinned people. | Seek medical advice to rule out the possibility of malignant melanoma. |
| **Onychatropia** | This is also know as atrophy—a wasting away of the nail plate. The nail loses its shine, shrinks, and sometimes even falls off. The problem can be caused by injury or internal disease, as well as nutritional or hereditary factors. | Handle this condition carefully. File the nail with a fine emery board and avoid using metal pushers, aggressive detergents, and soaps. New nails may grow back once any disease is cured. |
| **Onychauxis** | This is a condition where the nail plate becomes thick and clawlike, curving inward and sometimes extending over the tip of the finger. Often caused by trauma, it pinches the nail bed painfully and may need surgery to ease the pain. A very common condition, which usually occurs on toenails but can appear on fingernails too. | Often hereditary, it can also be caused by an imbalance or infection. While there is no permanent solution for this condition, filing and buffing the nail will reduce the thickness. Chronic onychauxis may require medical intervention. |
| **Paronychia** | Also called a "whitlow," this chronic infection of the nail tissue surrounding the nail results in redness, inflammation, and tenderness. Caused by a bacterial or yeast infection, it can occur at the base of the nail, around the whole nail, or on the tips of the fingers. You will be more prone to these problems if you pull your hangnails, suck your thumbs, or bite your nails. | Having your hands in water for extended periods of time also increases the risk of infection, so wear gloves and get medical advice for appropriate treatment. |

| | | |
|---|---|---|
| **Pseudomonas** | This bacterial infection occurs between the natural nail plate and the nail bed. In some cases it occurs between an artificial nail coating and the natural nail plate, especially if worn for extended periods without allowing the natural nail to breathe. The infection thrives in moist dark places, feeding off dead tissue and bacteria in the nail plate.<br><br>Usually the darker the discoloration, the further into the nail layers the bacteria has traveled. Once treated, it will take several months for the stain to grow out. | Always dry your hands thoroughly, as any additional moisture levels allow these bacteria to flourish. Try applying one drop of tea tree oil onto the affected area or soak in a 5 percent solution several times a day for a few days. An infected nail needs to be analyzed; depending on the cause, an antifungal or antibacterial remedy might be applied. If severe, consult a dermatologist. |
| **Psoriasis** | This skin condition is characterized by reddish dry spots and patches covered with silvery scales. When psoriasis affects the nail plate, the nail becomes pitted and dry and may change color and separate from the nail bed. If severe, the nail plate may disintegrate completely. | If psoriasis affects your nails, consult a dermatologist. |
| **Pterygium** | This common condition describes the abnormal growth of the cuticle over the nail plate. It is usually caused by trauma to the matrix and may even result in the loss of the nail. | Never try to remove the Pterygium yourself; consult a doctor for advice and treatment. |
| **Separation from the nail bed** | When the nail separates from the nail bed, the cause may be trauma or a thyroid disorder, but most often, the condition is unknown. | Carefully trim away the separated nail and seek medical advice. |

# SKIN SOLUTIONS

The skin on the fingers, hands, and arms is prone to many problems—from allergies to warts. Treating them correctly can prevent spreading and discomfort.

| Problem | Symptoms | Solution |
|---|---|---|
| **Itching** | Generalized itching may be an allergic reaction to a medication, cosmetic, or skincare product. Apply cold compresses and see a dermatologist to track down the source. If your eyelids are itchy, you may have a contact allergy to either latex or nickel, or to the formaldehyde in the polish on your nails. | Switching to a formaldehyde-free formula should clear it up. |
| **Rough, chapped hands** | Often caused by exposure to cold weather, for instance. Another cause of chapped and dry skin is repeated washing of the hands with harsh detergents, which can further contribute to cracks or fissures. Dry, chapped skin can also signal the first signs of a possible vitamin A deficiency. | Moisturize your hands after every wash and protect them from water and cleaning products. Try increasing your intake of vitamin A and use a rich moisturizing cream before going to bed. |

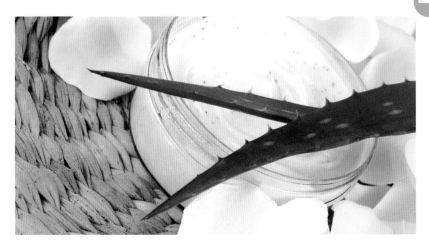

| | | |
|---|---|---|
| **Eczema** | Eczema, also called dermatitis, is a general term meaning inflammation of the skin, characterized by redness, pain, or itching. A lot of things can lead to dermatitis, including allergies, irritation, extreme dryness, and genetic factors.<br><br>Contact dermatitis or eczema is caused by a reaction to certain substances that touch the skin. The skin becomes red and itchy, and tiny blisters may develop. Sometimes these tiny blisters form large blisters that break, scale, and crust over. Harsh detergents, chemicals, and poisonous plants are often the culprits. | Applying a nonprescription steroid cream like hydrocortisone, together with an anti-itching lotion like calamine, as often as possible will help reduce the rash. Sweating can also irritate the rash, so avoid strenuous exercise if your skin has flared up. If you can't identify the allergy-causing agent, the next thing you need to do is to lessen the allergic inflammatory response. Use a hypoallergenic soap to clean the area everyday, apply a lubricating cream after washing, avoid stress, eat right, get adequate sleep, and don't exert yourself. All this helps to minimize flare-ups. Eczema is easier to control than it is to cure. |
| **Allergies** | Skin can be bothered by cosmetics, clothing, chemicals, air pollution, diet, or health changes. Reactions appear as allergic swelling, blemishes, hives, local irritation, or rashes. | The best way to handle contact allergies is to avoid the offending substance. So protect yourself by being aware of what you touch. Remember that often you can have contact with an allergen but the allergic reaction shows up in another area of your body, so wearing gloves is the best defense. |
| **Warts** | Warts are skin growths caused by a viral infection in the top layer of the skin or mucus membranes. The virus responsible belongs to the group called papillomavirus. Warts are usually skin-colored and rough-textured, though some can be dark, smooth, and flat. Wart viruses are spread by touch, but they can take several months before the wart gets big enough to be visible. | Most warts will eventually disappear and scratching and picking will cause them to spread. If an over-the-counter preparation doesn't work, seek medical help. |

# HEALTHY HANDS

Pay special attention to your hands when tending to your beauty needs. Exfoliate them regularly to remove dead skin cells and slather on hand creams. Use a preparation containing sunscreens while outdoors.

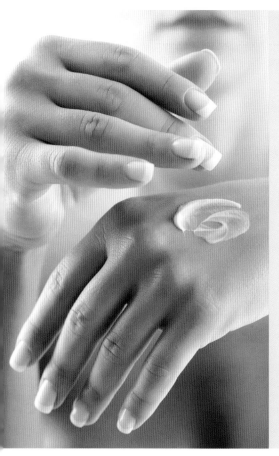

- Apply hand cream every time you wash your hands. Keep tubs of hand cream beside the sink or basin.
- Always wear rubber gloves. Plunging unprotected hands and nails into soapy water or household chemicals is like going into the sun without sunblock. Cotton-lined rubber gloves are best to absorb excess moisture.
- Exfoliate the backs of your hands whenever you use a scrub or exfoliator on your body or face.
- Massage your hands with hand cream whenever you have a few spare moments. Use the first finger and the thumb of the opposite hand and work in small circles, moving from the tips of your fingers to your wrist.
- Finger exercises can prevent Occupational Overuse Syndrome (OOS), formerly known as Repetitive Strain Injury (RSI). This syndrome occurs from constant, repetitive actions such as typing. Exercise your fingers by clenching them into a ball, then slowly release them and stretch the fingers out. Rotate your wrists in circular movements.
- Use a hand cream with full-spectrum sun filters to protect your hands from sun damage and age-spots.

# 7 steps to healthy hands

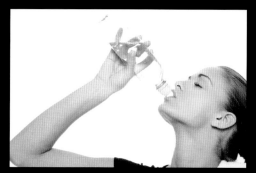

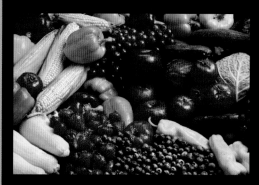

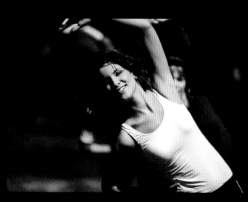

- **Drink** at least six glasses of pure water a day to keep the skin moisturized inside and out.
- **Eat right**. Choose foods that are healthy and as close to "natural" as possible. Vary the type of fruit and vegetables.
- Get the **sleep** your body needs—usually six to eight hours every night.
- **Wear sunscreen** and protective clothing to avoid overexposing your skin to the elements. Some sunshine is necessary, but today's suntan is tomorrow's aging skin.
- **Avoid temperature extremes** and harsh detergents; instead, wash with mild cleansers. As a normal skin function, sweat and sebaceous glands routinely rid the body of toxins and wastes.
- **Protect your hands** with moisturizing creams, sunscreen, or the appropriate gloves when you are exposing your hands to abrasive substances or environmental elements.
- **Exercise**. When you are faced with repetitive tasks, take regular time out to stretch and wiggle your fingers, wrists, hands, and arms to maintain a normal range of movement.

# JOINT FLEXIBILITY AND MOVEMENT

Whether swinging a tennis racket or typing, human fingers, wrists, and arms are designed for movement. With time and overuse, however, all of us are affected by stiffness and aches resulting from overuse.

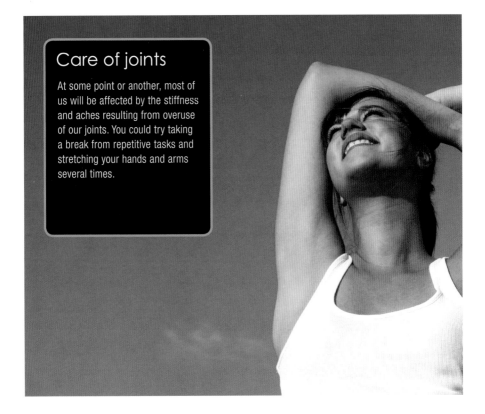

## Care of joints

At some point or another, most of us will be affected by the stiffness and aches resulting from overuse of our joints. You could try taking a break from repetitive tasks and stretching your hands and arms several times.

| Problem | Symptoms | Solution |
|---------|----------|----------|
| **Occupational Overuse Syndrome— OOS** | This is the term given to a range of conditions characterized by discomfort or persistent pain in muscles, tendons, and other soft tissues. These conditions are usually caused or aggravated by unsuitable working conditions involving repetitive or forceful movements, or the maintenance of constrained or awkward postures. OOS is also known as Repetitive Strain Injury (RSI). Some of the problems that can be caused by OOS are: **Carpal Tunnel Syndrome** Pressure on the median nerve in the wrist, which causes numbness and tingling in the fingers and hand. **Tenosynovitis** Pain and swelling of the tendons, often in the hands and wrists. **Epicondylitis** Pain and tenderness of the muscles and tendons around the elbow. **Static Muscle Strain** Occurs when muscles are used to keep part of the body still for long periods of time. This can cause pain and stiffness in muscles, often in the shoulders, neck, and forearms. Symptoms of OOS often include swelling, numbness, restricted movement, and weakness in or around muscles and tendons of the back, neck, shoulders, elbows, wrists, hands, or fingers. It may become difficult to hold objects or tools in the hands, affecting your ability to function at work and at home. | Avoid movements that cause pain and consult a doctor. |
| **Carpal Tunnel Syndrome** | Caused when one of the nerves leading from the wrist to the hand is compressed as it passes through the carpal tunnel, a space in the wrist through which tendons that flex the fingers also pass. The pressure causes pain and loss of some use of the hand. This condition mainly affects people who use their fingers a lot, like typists, housewives, or pianists. Symptoms include pain, tingling, and numbness in the thumb, index finger, and middle finger of the affected hand. Pain tends to be worse at night, getting gradually worse over a period of weeks. | Avoid movements that cause pain and consult a doctor. |

# CARING FOR LONG NAILS

While long nails and nail art are not always sensible or attractive, everyone has different tastes and lifestyles, and long nails and nail adornment may very well fit into yours.

If you choose to have long nails, learn how to use your fingers; get into the habit of using them as if you have just applied a fresh coat of nail polish. The more trauma nails suffer, the more likely the tips will break. People are often surprised at how easily nails break, yet few realize the damage began days, even weeks, earlier.

Long nails and pointed nails are, by nature, weaker than "normally" shaped nails, so they require special attention. Several coats of nail hardener will help to minimize chipping and peeling of the nail enamel. The trick is to find something that protects and moisturizes. Nail hardeners with nylon fibers can be very effective.

General reminders for long nails are:

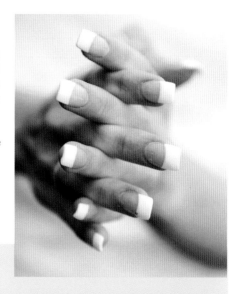

- Avoid using nail tips to untie knots or loosen shoelaces.
- Use the sides of your fingers to open car doors.
- Do not dial the telephone with your fingers; use a pen or pencil.
- Use your knuckles to press buttons, such as those in elevators.
- Use a knife or razor to open boxes and packages, not your nails; nails were not designed to be used as screwdrivers, apple corers, or hors d'oeuvre utensils.
- Use the pads of your fingers rather than your nails while typing.
- Always use rubber gloves when handling household cleaners or bleach, because these quickly dry out your nails, leaving them brittle.
- When putting on pantyhose or stockings, keep your index fingers turned under and use the middle portion of the thumb to pull them up. This not only saves your nails, but increases the lifespan of your pantyhose.

# Pro tips for nail-biters

Chronic nail-biting deforms
the nail plate and damages the
tissue surrounding it, resulting
in unattractive nails and the
introduction of bacteria that may
cause illness and minor, but
permanent, nail deformities. Regular
manicures help nail-biters become
more conscientious of their nails
and encourage them to stop biting.

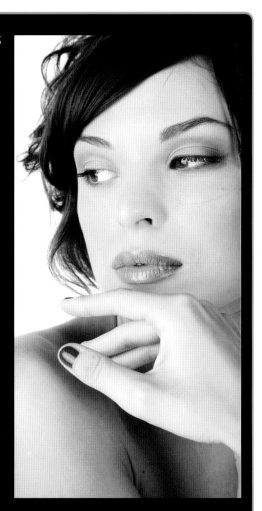

- Devote 10 minutes every day
  to caring for your nails; as they
  start to look prettier, you will be
  more inclined to want to stop
  biting them.
- Try one of the anti-biting lotions
  on the market. Having stopped
  for a couple of weeks, your longer
  nails will give you the incentive to
  keep up the good work.
- Having short nails does not mean
  you cannot wear nail polish;
  even short nails look better with
  an application of clear or pale
  colored polish.
- Consider wearing artificial
  nails or properly applied nail
  enhancements for a while, so
  your nails have a chance to
  grow underneath. Even the most
  determined nail-biters have
  trouble gnawing their way through
  them! A few weeks might be all
  you need to break the habit.
- Carry an emery board with you
  at all times, so you can instantly
  smooth away straggly edges that
  tempt you to bite.

# GALLERY

There are so many different style choices possible; the only limit is in your knowledge of what can be achieved. The

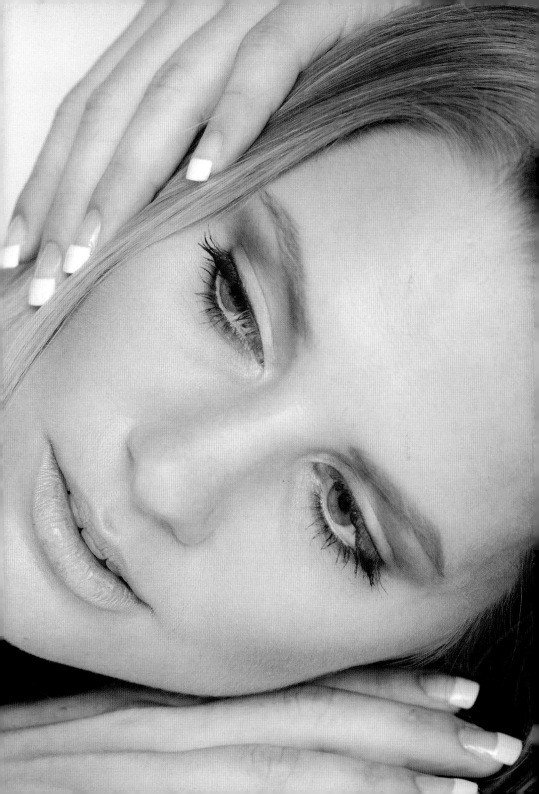

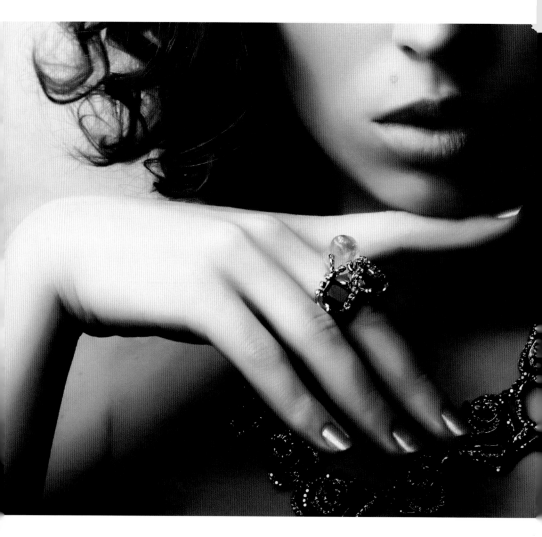

**↑ Sophisticated pink**
This subtle pink complements most skin tones
and suits a glamorous black outfit.

**↘ Bright pink**
This brighter shade is appropriate
for both day and evening looks.

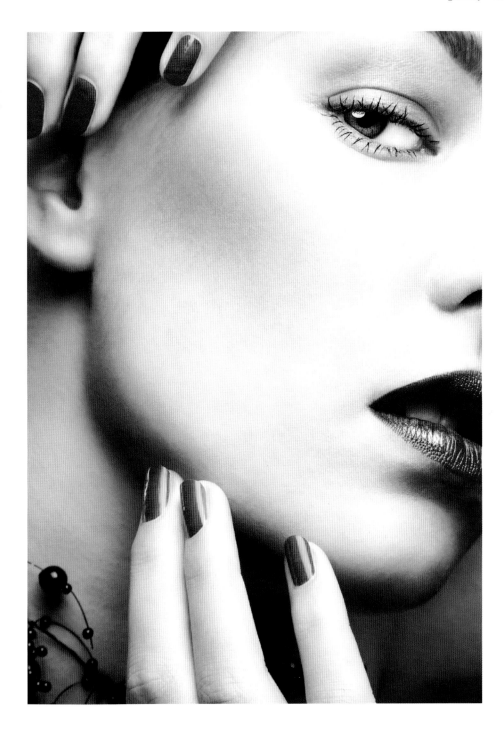

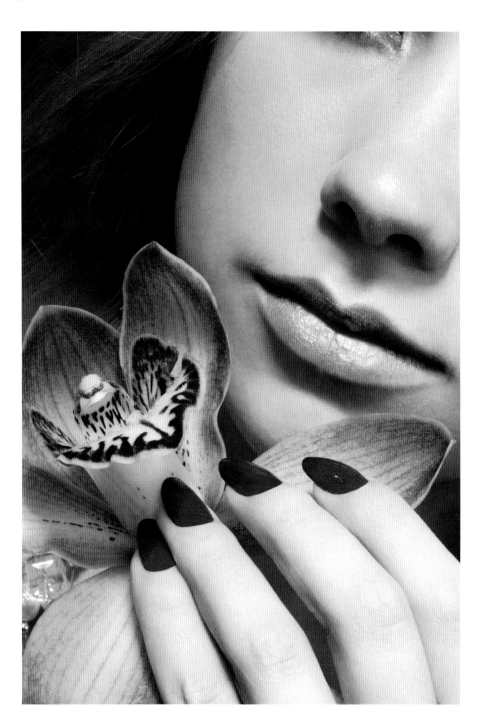

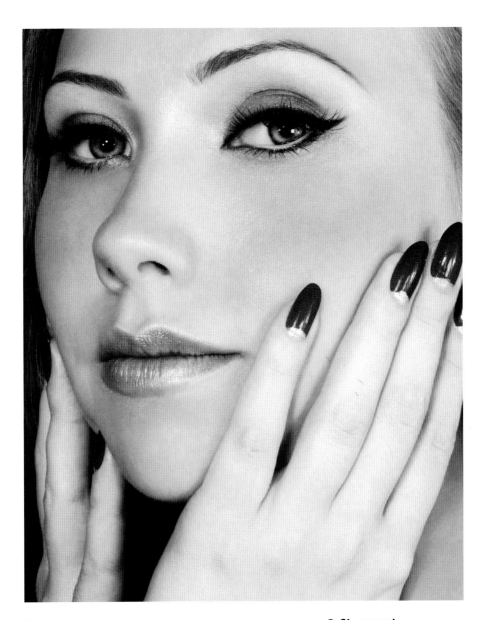

**⊙ Fuchsia**
Designed to distract, a bright, vibrant
fuchsia shade says "look at me."

**⊙ Cherry red**
Hotter than pink, but not as saucy
as a deep red color.

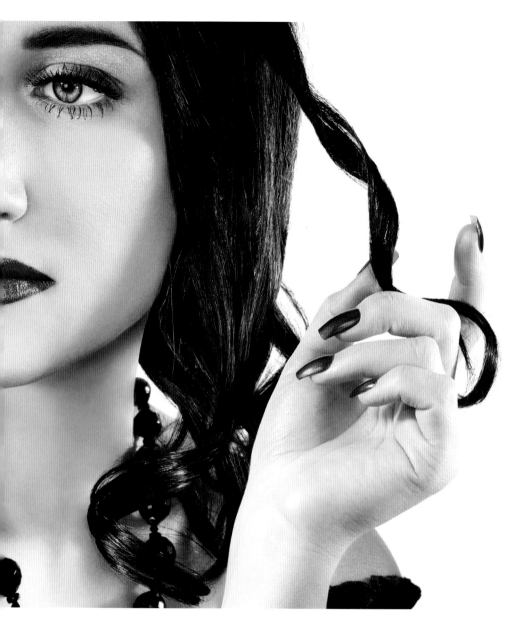

**⬆ Deep red**

A classic, timeless color for
evening and day.

**↑ Burnt copper**
A summery version of the classic deep red.

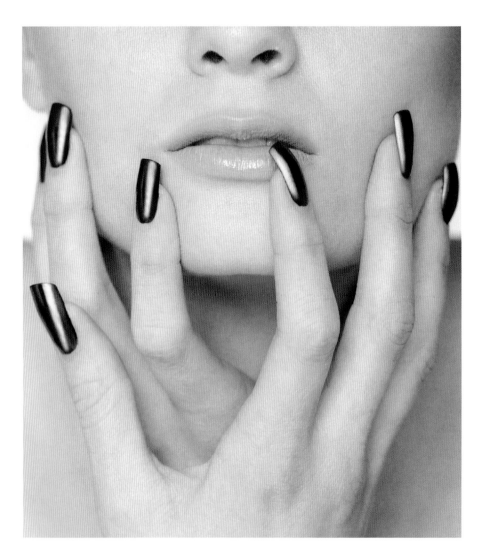

**⬆ Dark metallic gray**

Ultramodern and chic, dark
metallic gray looks good on long
talons for an evening out.

**➡ Silver**

Cool and refreshing,
silver is suitable for both
winter and summer.

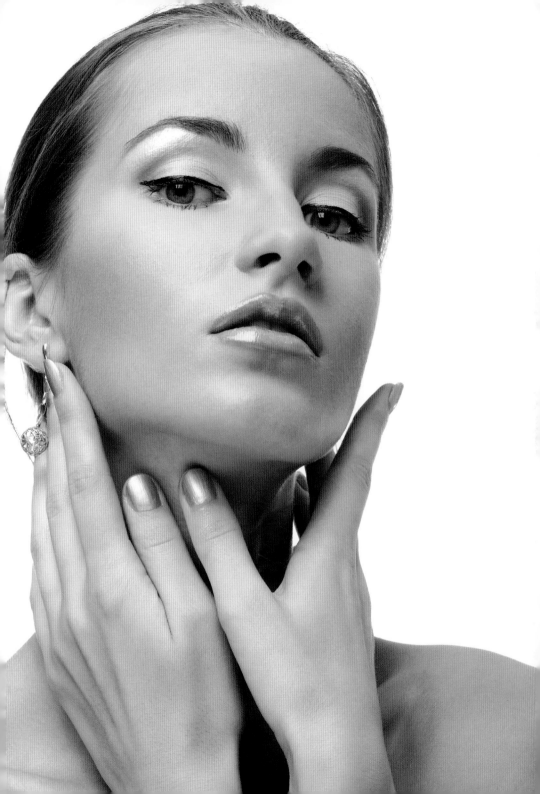

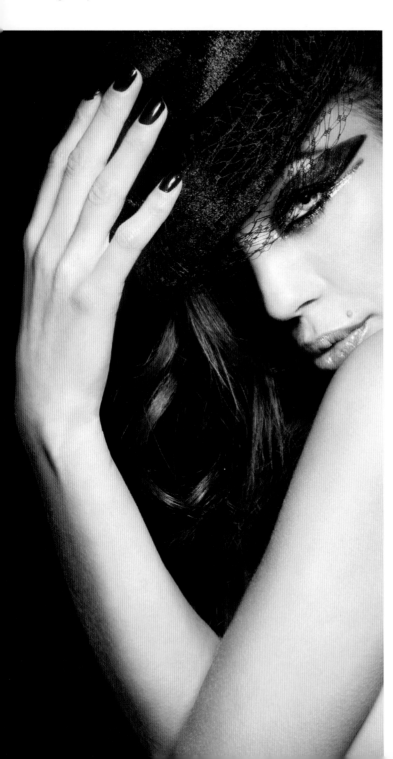

**◐ Black**
The color of rock chicks, chocolate and black polish were popular shades during the 1990s.

**◑ Black**
A great base for nail art, especially bright-colored polka dots.

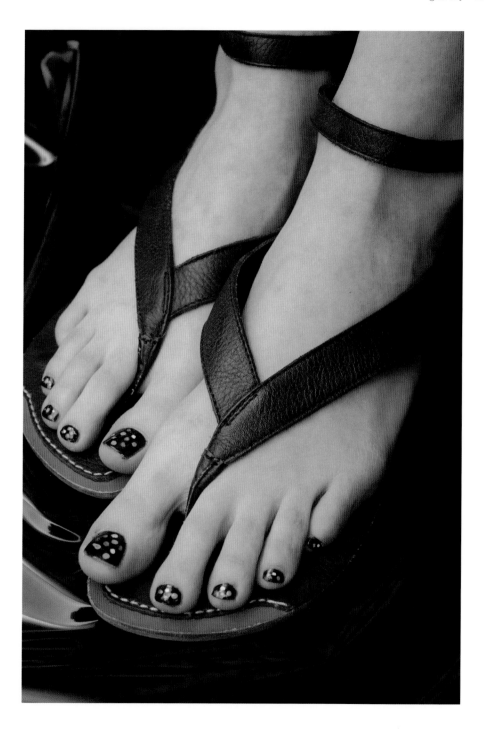

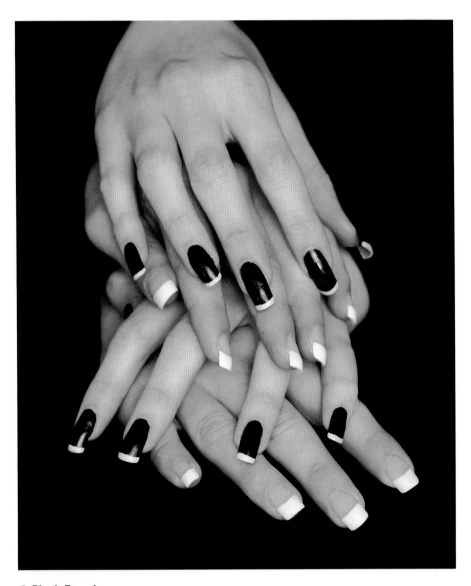

**↑ Black French**

Experiment with the traditional
French manicure by mixing black
together with different color tips.

**➲ Black**

Can be ultracool and sexy if your
nails are not too long.

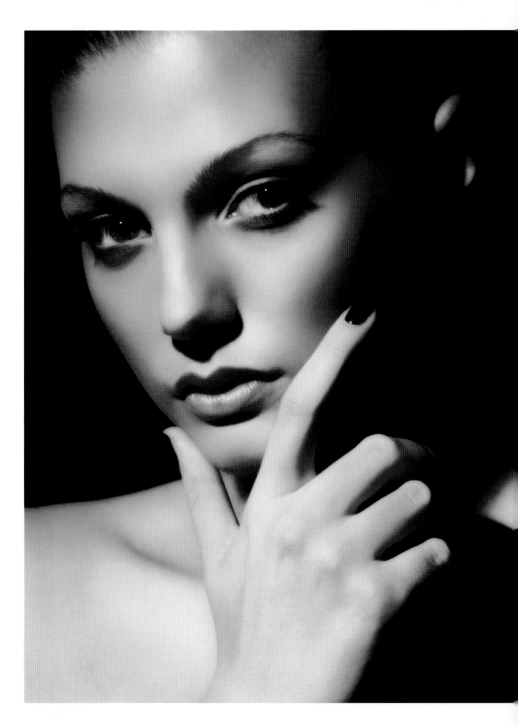

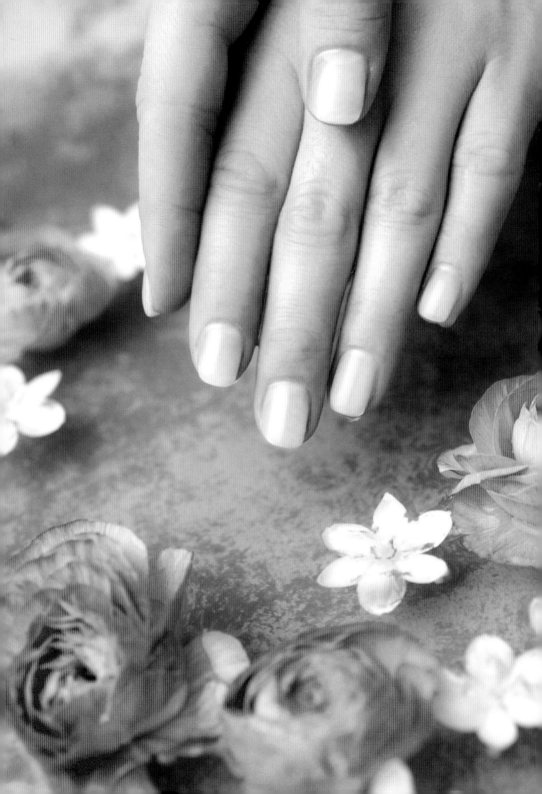

## ⬅ French manicure

Suitable for the office or an evening out.
The French manicure speaks volumes about
the pride you take in your appearance.

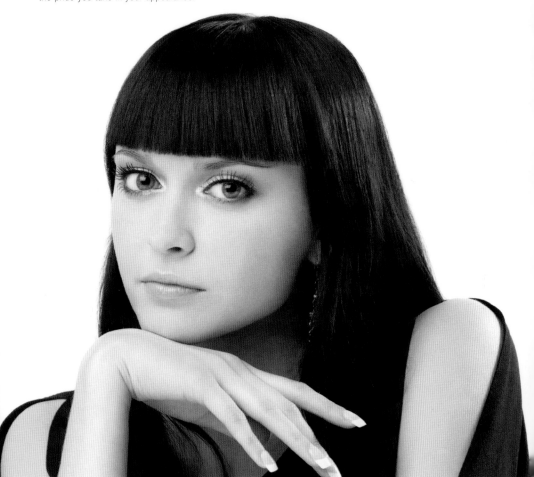

## ⬆ French manicure

Worn with longer nails, this can
look really feminine.

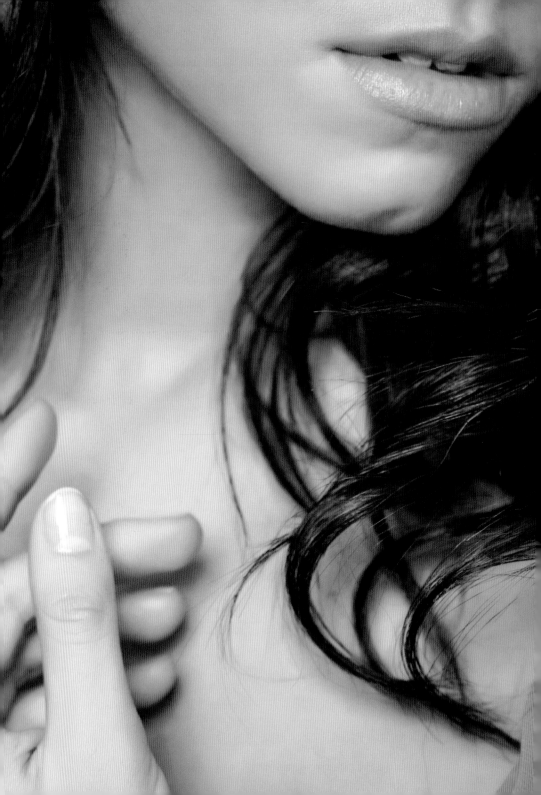

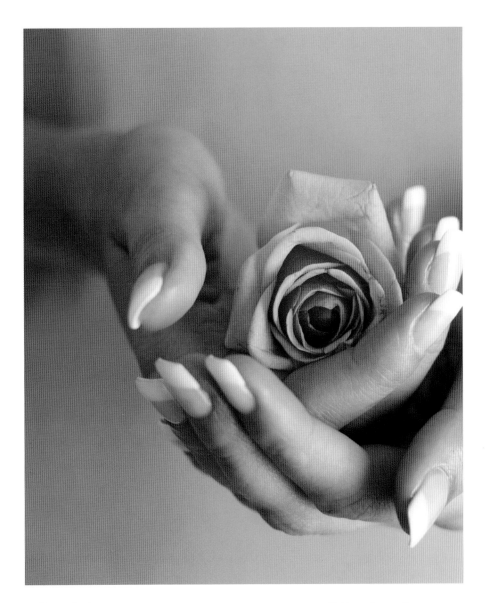

### ◐ Natural gloss
Just a hint of polish—subtle
enough for the office, but enough
to say you care about your nails.

### ◑ French manicure
Looks good on your natural nails
but also perfect for acrylics.

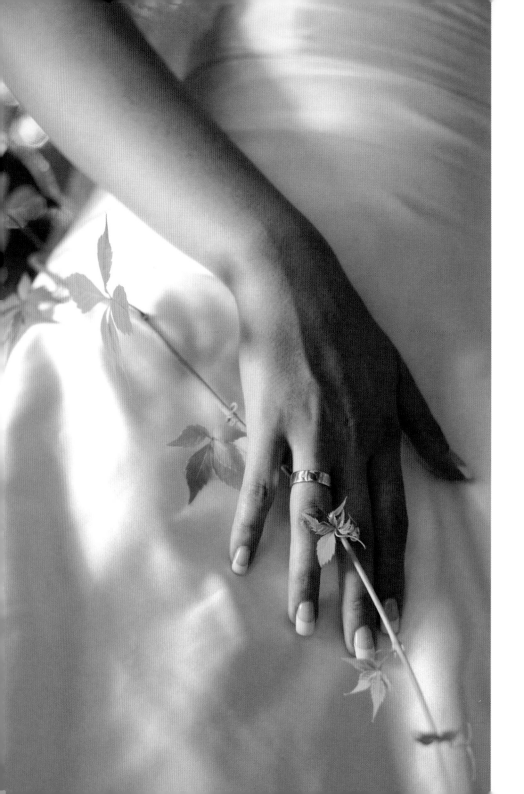

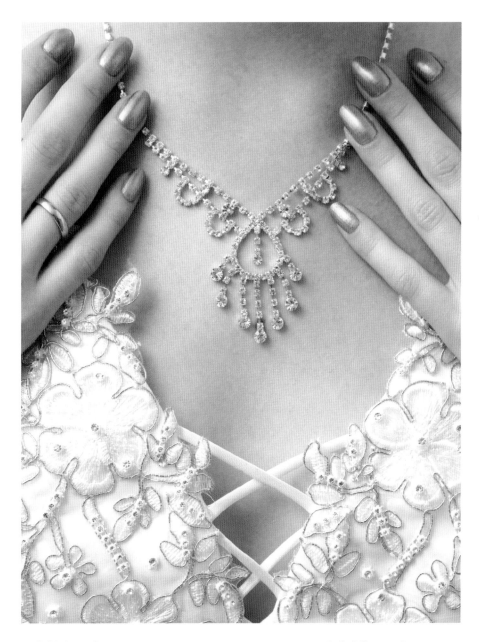

### ◑ Bridal manicure
Subtle but beautiful and ultrafeminine—this French manicure won't draw attention away from your dress.

### ⬆ Subtle peach
Complements ivories and golds.

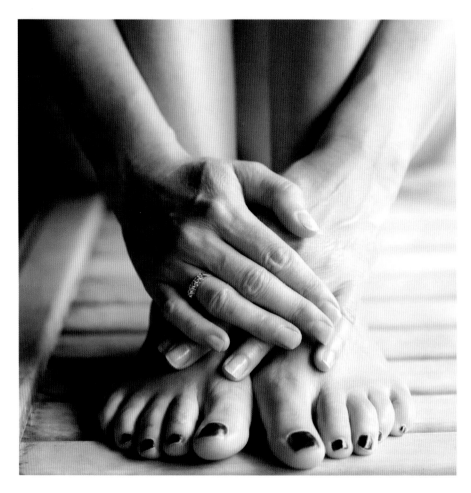

**➊ Red/brown toes**
Perfect for open toe sandals in the summer months.

**➋ Natural toes**
Subtle but healthy-looking. Ideal for long summer days spent in open toe sandals.

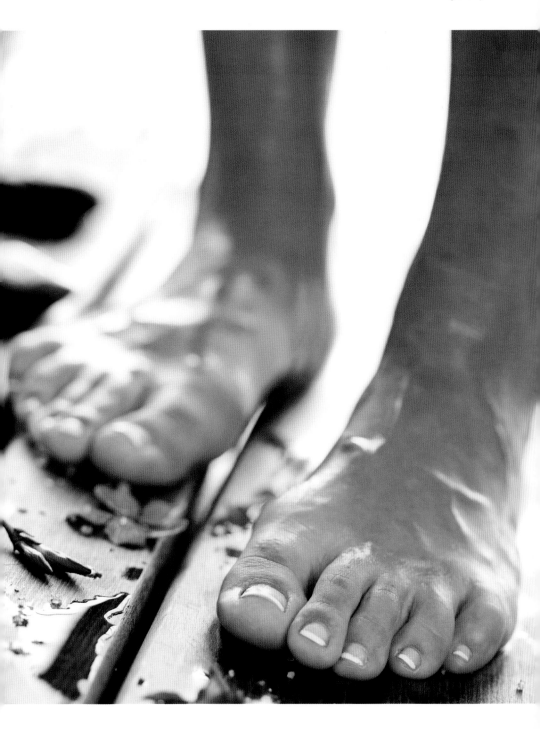

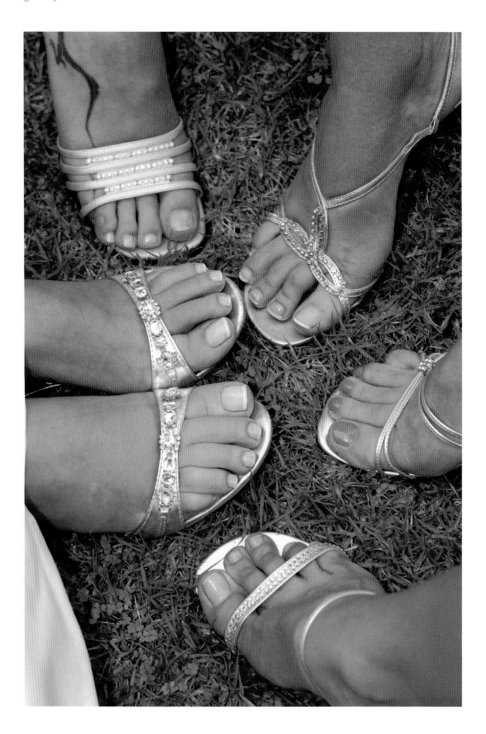

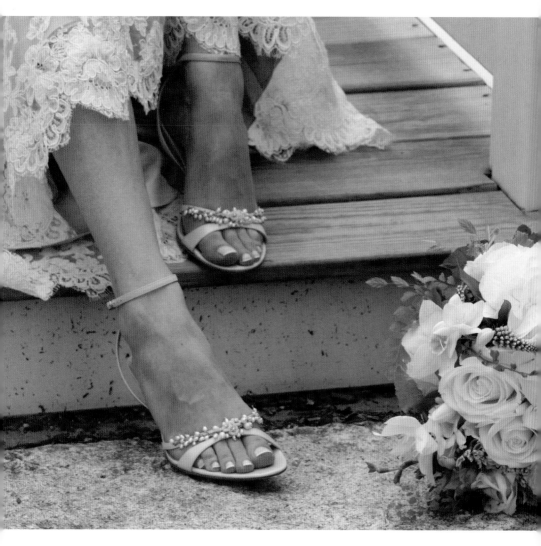

### ◉ Bridal pedicure

Whether you are the bride or her
grandmother, if you're wearing
open toe sandals to a wedding,
polish is a must.

### ◉ Bridal pedicure

Natural looking, elegant toes are
best for a wedding.

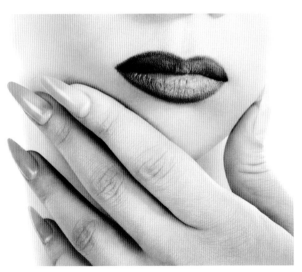

### ➲ Nail art
Transfers are very quick and easy to use.

### ⬆ Acrylics
Long, pointed acrylics are quite a strong look.

### ⬇ False nails
These are very long and bold but many women love them—use with caution!

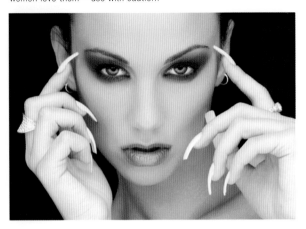

### ➲ Nail art
Subtle transfers in white look good on a pale pink.

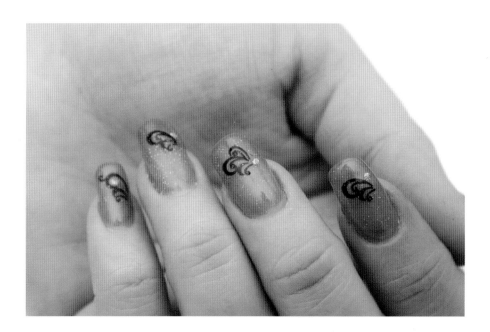

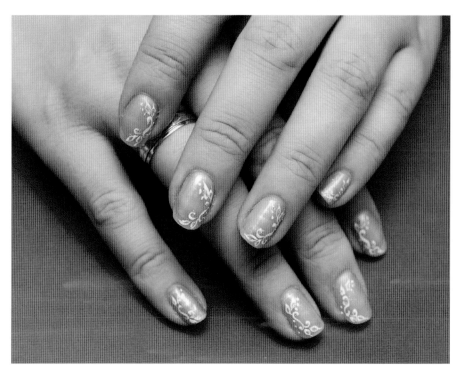

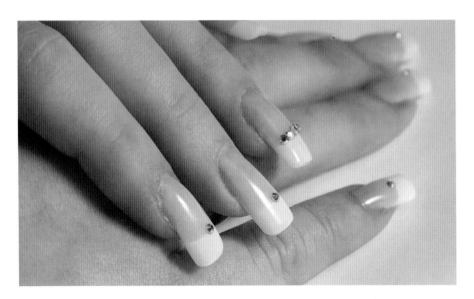

### ⬆ Nail art

Gems and diamanté are very pretty
on French acrylics.

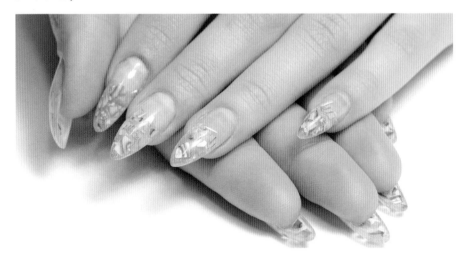

### ⬆ Nail art

Be aware of all the different styles available for
your nail art and don't let yourself be limited
by a narrow range of colors.

### ⬇ Nail art

Superlong, pointy talons are one of
the options out there—some women
love them!

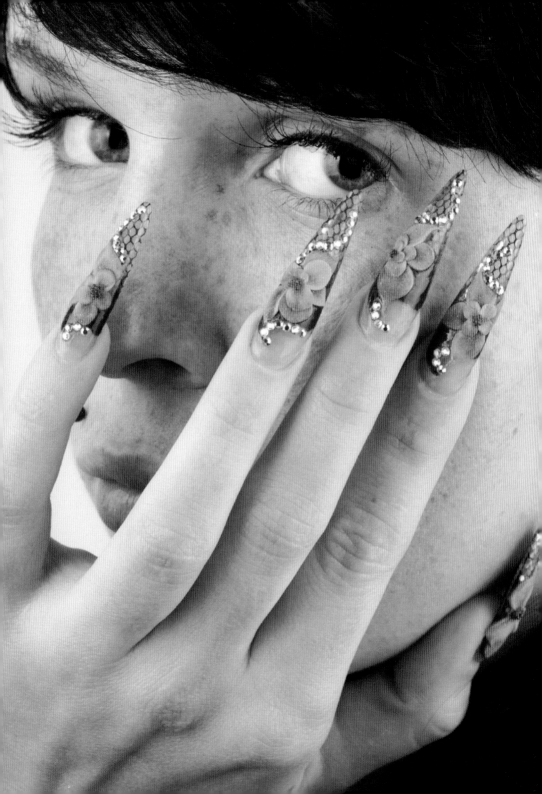

# TAKING IT FURTHER

## Getting started

To become a nail technician, formal training is essential and students will need to take a cosmetology program. These courses are available at technical colleges, cosmetology schools, beauty schools, community colleges, and vocational training centers. Each country has different requirements, but regardless of where you are in the world, training is usually carried out in a college environment, and a set number of hours of practical learning and application must be achieved before completing a practical exam. Courses usually cover the following: science of nail technology, manicuring and pedicuring, nail treatments, nail wraps, acrylic and gel nails, nail art, bacteriology and sanitation, anatomy and physiology of the skin and nail, product chemistry, hand and arm massage, the business of nail technology, professional etiquette, salesmanship, and shop management.

Certification in safety, hygiene, and professional techniques is also essential if you intend to enter the workplace. Training programs can take as little as a few months or they can run over an entire year. They teach nail hygiene, safety, shaping, coloring, and more. There are also all sorts of top-up courses available to extend your qualifications and knowledge. Once you're qualified, you'll be able to work in beauty salons and spas, or even start your own business and look for clients on your own. "Post-graduate" training services are sometimes available through nail companies—product manufacturers and suppliers provide invaluable input in terms of chemicals, products and their usage—so make good use of them to advance your knowledge and gain a thorough understanding of their products and services. They are also very useful for keeping up-to-date with all the new technological advances.

## Going professional

A hard-working independent technician should be able to build a successful business and thriving clientele. Usually the most sought-after positions are in high-end salons and spas; these jobs are usually reserved for the more experienced and skilled workers. There are many career paths that you can choose from according to your particular strengths and interests, from apprentice work for an established salon to running a home-based salon or a mobile salon, renting a booth in an established salon, teaching, working on cruise ships, or through all-inclusive holiday packages, or even purchasing an existing franchise. Rates of pay will also vary—some nail technicians are paid an hourly wage and many salons also pay sales commission, but that will all depend on the salon owner.

Working from home, starting with just a few clients, some word-of-mouth advertising, and a lot of hard work, can start off a hugely successful business in a matter of months. While the setting up can be as inexpensive or as expensive as you want it to be, the benefits of not having to work restricted hours can be a real advantage if you have a family. Working from home is a practical solution for a lot of people as the low overheads, no commuting, and flexible hours far outweigh the negatives, which include having strangers in your home and working alone.

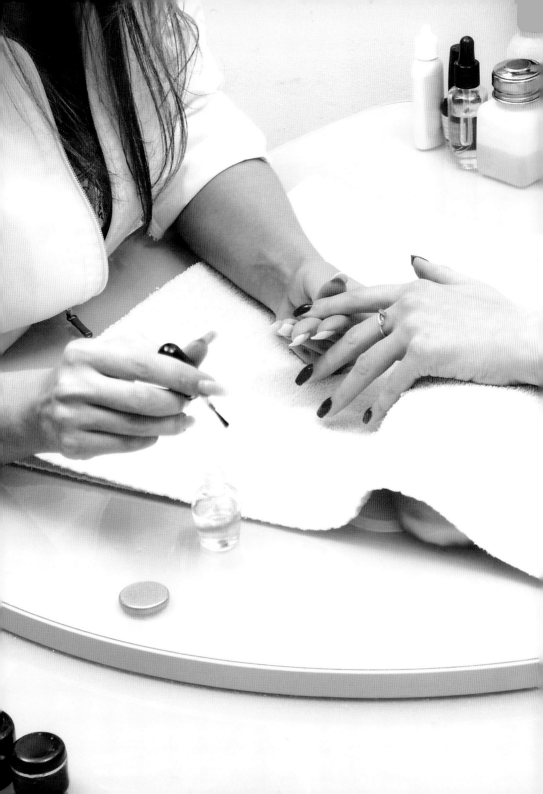

# SUPPLIERS

## www.handsdown.co.za

A broad spectrum of products for every aspect of the beauty industry including professional products for the qualified nail technician.

## www.tweezerman.com

Offer all sorts of tweezers and nailcare tools with a lifetime sharpening guarantee.

## www.jessicacosmetics.com

A great resource for professional products, their Custom Colors are formaldehyde, toluene, and DBP free (dibutyl phthalate is a commonly used plasticizer). Also, interactive color selector, advice on your specific nail type, and lots of tips and pointers.

## www.sallyhansen.com

Lots of tips and pointers on nail colors and treatments, artificial nails, as well as hand and foot care.

## www.feetforlife.org

A chiropody website with lots of information about healthy feet, including advice on shoes, foot problems, and how to maintain healthy feet.

## www.goodfeet.com

A great site to help you locate arch supports and orthoses, as well as cushion and comfort shoes.

## www.dreamyfeet.co.uk

Good source for products and information relating to foot pain.

## www.footcaredirect.com

Useful information on anything to do with the study and treatment of foot, heel, and ankle conditions.

## www.cir-safety.org

If you have any concerns about the ingredients in nail products and treatments, this is well worth checking out—they have lists of ingredients, as well as advice on possible allergic reactions or signs of poisoning.

## www.youngnails.com

Step-by-step tutorials online and a host of products from specialized tools, and colored acrylic powders to acrylic nail art supplies.

## www.opi.com

Everything you need for color including a try-this-on guide, as well as Suzi's beauty blog with lots of style and fashion tips, quick-tip videos, fashion pointers, and diagnostic advice.

## www.orlybeauty.com

Products galore including natural-looking nail products for men and deterrents for nail-biters, with online lessons and more.

## www.drscholls.com

Everything to do with healthy feet and the care of your feet, including a diagnostic guide on how to recognize foot problems and practical advice on how to solve them.

## www.cbsexquisite.com

Supplies for nails, pedicures, facial steamers, airbrush supplies, waxing supplies, skincare, and spa and all relevant furnishings.

## www.essie.com

Fabulous fashion nail products.

## www.atyourfingertips.org.uk

Nail salon supplies including nail art, accessories, tools, rhinestones, tips, gel and acrylic systems, airbrushing supplies, IBD soak-off gels, acrylic liquids and powders, daylight lamps, polishes, and a whole lot more besides.

## www.trind.com

A wide selection of nail treatments, products, and manicure tools.

## www.idonails.com

The supply source for everything you'll need to set up a salon from furniture and empty containers to adhesives, abrasives, implements, acrylic accessories, and all related products.

## www.gel-nails.com

Online catalog of gel nail kits, nail art supplies from rhinestones to transfers, dappen dishes to drills and drill bits, and all the equipment like forms, tips, tools, and more.

## www.beautydesign.com

A great resource for setting up from furniture to layout and design, plus all the eqiuipment you might need.

## www.nails-r-us.com

Salon supplies, tools, accessories, and preparations.

## www.nsinails.com

Tutorial videos, a wide selection of professional products, and access to all sorts of technical information, provided you're a registered member.

# TERMINOLOGY

## Acid-based

A term that refers to primers that contain methacrylic acid.

## Acid-free

Primers that contain absolutely no acid components.

## Acrylonitrile-butadine-styrene (ABS)

A thermoplastic, from which most pre-formed tips are made.

## Apex

The highest point on the nail plate.

## Breathing zone

A one-meter sphere that surrounds your head, from which you draw all the air you breathe.

## Built-up tips

Oval paper or metal inserted under the nail before acrylic is painted on and allowed to set; finally, the tip is filed to the chosen shape.

## Carpal tunnel

A small passage in the wrist that houses the nerve that runs from the fingers into the arm.

## C-curve

The curve of the nail from wall to wall, as seen from the tip.

## Distal

The furthest attached end of the nail.

## Effleurage

A stroking massage movement.

## Film formers

Ingredients used to create a continuous coating on the nail plate—like nitrocellulose.

# Flexibility

The property that allows a substance to bend without cracking or shattering.

# Free edge

The part of the nail that extends beyond the fingertip.

# Gel nails

Created by applying layers of acrylic gel to the nail; the layers combine and harden to form a solid, natural-looking nail enhancement.

# Gelling

Partial, premature polymerization of monomer liquid, UV gel, wraps, or adhesives, while still in their original container.

# Guardian seal

A fold of skin pushing up against the nail plate that protects and prevents bacterial and chemical penetration.

# Lateral

To the side.

# Mix ratio

The correct mixture of powder and liquid to create nail extensions.

# Overlay

A thin coating applied to the natural nail to strengthen and protect.

# Petrissage

A compressive massage movement.

# Pre-tailoring

Adjustment and customization of the tip before fitting.

# Proximal

The nearest attached end.

# Smile line

The natural nail area where the nail leaves the nail plate; in a nail extension this is a clean white line that defines the tip.

# Stop point

The thicker part of the tip just below the stress area where the free edge will fit.

# Stress area

The area of the nail that has to take the most wear and tear.

# Volatile

Quickly evaporating.

# Wraps

A term used in fiberglass systems for the material used to overlay and reinforce the natural nail.

# INDEX

# CREDITS

pp1, 3: Corbis © Chris Collins/Corbis; p8: Corbis © Bettmann/Corbis; p10: Getty © George Marks; p11: Getty © Fox Photos; pp12–13: Getty © Rob Goldman; pp14, 15: Istock; pp18, 19, 20: Shutterstock; p60: Istock; p23: Shutterstock; p25: Istock; pp29, 35: Shutterstock; pp36, 37, 43, 45: Istock; pp56–57: Shutterstock; p61: Istock; pp63, 64, 65, 66, 67: Shutterstock; p69: Istock; pp70, 73, 75, 76, 84, 85: Shutterstock; pp86, 93: Istock; pp98, 99, 101, 102, 103 *top*: Shutterstock; p103 *below*: Istock; p108: Shutterstock; p109: Getty © Studio MPM; pp110, 114, 117: Shutterstock; p119: Istock; p131: Shutterstock; p144: Istock; p145: Shutterstock; p150: Corbis © Underwood & Underwood/corbis; p151 *top right, below left*: Corbis © Condé Nast Archive/Corbis; p151 *below right*: Istock; p152 *left*: Getty © Fox Photos; p152 *right*: Shutterstock; p153: Corbis © Steve Schapiro/Corbis; p154: Shutterstock; p155: Istock; p156: Shutterstock; pp158, 160, 161, 162: Istock; pp165, 167: Shutterstock; pp169, 171: Istock; p175: Shutterstock; p177: Getty © AFP/Getty Images; p178: Istock; p199: Shutterstock; p200: Istock; pp202, 204: Shutterstock; pp208, 210: Istock; p211 *top*: Shutterstock, *center, below*: Istock; p212: Shutterstock; pp 214, 215, 218, 219, 220, 221, 222: Istock; pp223, 225: Shutterstock; pp226, 229, 230, 231, 232, 233, 234, 235, 236: Istock; p237: Shutterstock; pp238, 239, 240, 241, 242, 243: Istock; p247: Shutterstock; p257: Istock.

**All other images are the copyright of Quintet Publishing Ltd. While every effort has been made to credit contributors, Quintet Publishing would like to apologize should there have been any omissions or errors—and would be pleased to make the appropriate correction for future editions of the book.**

## Acknowledgments

Special thanks to everyone who helped me with the project: trainer and nail technician Romilda Strijdom for her fastidious attention to detail and for patiently going through each and every step for the camera in spite of personal dramas; Yolanda Bekker and Lindiwe Ngubeni of Young Nails who showed us their acrylic nail art techniques, shared their products, and allowed us to invade their salon; Trevor Feinauer of Smartbuy for loaning us heaps of equipment and products and for sharing his endless knowledge; Colleen O'Connell at Handsdown Distribution for lots of technical advice, products, technical savvy, and equipment; Jessica Nails for supplying us with products; the team at Quintet; my husband/photographer Patrick Toselli for his support and hard work; and of course, my incredible back-up team—all my boys! Thank you.

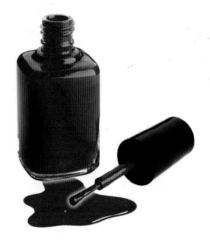